Best of the World Recipes

Although these recipes have been adapted to healthier alternatives with reduced oil and no animal products, for optimum health it is recommended that you eliminate salt, oil and sugar (SOS) altogether. You will find pencil notations by me where this elimination is easy:

- Substitute a good homemade vegetable broth for oil (or water when sautéing onions and/or vegetables.)
- Substitute apple sauce for oil in baked goods and pesto sauces.
- Substitute Benson's "Table Tasty" for salt.
- Substitute Date Sugar for sweeteners and sugar.

Two of our favorite San Diego Restaurants are:
- *Purple Mint* - all vegan Vietnamese Bistro

- *Jyoti-Bihanga* – vegan neatloaf sandwich, daily vegan specials, soups and bowls.

- Veggie Grill

Love,
Bonie

The Best in the World IV

HEALTHFUL RECIPES FROM EXCLUSIVE
AND OUT-OF-THE-WAY RESTAURANTS

Edited by

Neal D. Barnard, M.D.

Copyright ©2014 by
Physicians Committee for Responsible Medicine
5100 Wisconsin Ave., Suite 400, Washington, DC 20016

.Book design: Doug Hall

ISBN-10: 1-935535-02-1
ISBN-13: 978-1-935535-02-7

First printing November 2014

10 9 8 7 6 5 4 3 2 1

Printed in Canada

Foreword

*I*f you are new to *The Best in the World* series, you are in for a treat. We have compiled some of the most delicious and most healthful recipes you could ever imagine, all coming from exclusive and out-of-the way restaurants from around the world.

Just as you're licking the garlic and truffle white bean dip from your fingers (the very best in Curaçao) and wondering if that really is Prosecco in the melon soup at Washington's La Tomate (of course it is!), you'll have to decide whether to drop in for Krystal's canelones de verduras in the Spanish island of Tenerife or sample the daal bati at the Imperial Palace in Rajkot, Gujarat. Or maybe you'd like to keep it simple with a pizza. But this is not just any pizza; in Pompeii, where Vesuvius blew its lid in AD 79, you'll still taste the heat in Zi Caterina's pizza Napolitano.

In cases where a chef might have been overly exuberant with olive oil or poured cheese over a dish, we have adjusted recipes to reduce the fat content and to make everything suitable for plant-based palates. Still, you'll taste the original flavors in every recipe, and I hope you enjoy them as much as we did in bringing them to you.

We want to thank the many people who brought this book to fruition, starting with the restaurateurs who lent their wonderful recipes. Shaina Chimes worked with the many restaurants and chefs, tracked down recipes, coordinated the careful recipe testing, and kept this project organized. Amber Green, R.D., and Susan Levin, M.S., R.D., handled the nutrient analyses and edited the recipes. Alexandra Georgiadis, Amanda Ethridge, Andrea Cimino, Anne Bunner, Annie Halsey, Aryenish Birdie, Bonnie MacLeod, Cammie Wolff, Clarissa Barton, Craig Ziskin, Dania DePas, Francesca Valente, Jamie Berger,

Jodie Hayward, Katie Vann, Kristie Sullivan, Lynn Maurer, Margaret Murray, Mallory Huff, Noah Gittell, Patrick Carr, Sara Howe, Shaina Chimes, Stacey Glaeser, Tess Maggio, and Zeeshan Ali tested the recipes, and Doug Hall turned these words into a work of art.

NEAL D. BARNARD, M.D.

Contents

Appetizers

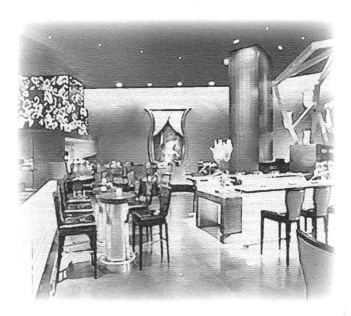

RED MISO EGGPLANT WITH CRISPY TOFU,
THAI BASIL, AND MINT

Izakaya, Borgata, Atlantic City, New Jersey

MAKES 3 SERVINGS

*I*f you can tear yourself away from the Borgata's gaming tables, Atlantic City's most chic casino hides a treasure. The Izakaya restaurant is truly clever in presentation, taste, and everything else.

2 baby eggplants, Japanese preferred
2 tablespoons salt
4 cups plus 3 tablespoons canola oil, divided
1 shallot, minced
2 ounces firm tofu, 1/2-inch cubes

2 tablespoons cornstarch
2 teaspoons minced garlic cloves
1/4 red finger chili pepper, thinly sliced
6 Thai basil leaves, chiffonade
4 mint leaves, chiffonade
3/4 cup chopped fresh cilantro

SAUCE (MAKES 8 OUNCES)

1 cup sake

1 1/2 teaspoons chili paste

1 cup mirin (Japanese sweet cooking wine)

1 ounce white miso paste

6 ounces red miso paste

1/4 cup apple cider vinegar

Cut the ends off of each eggplant. Slice eggplant lengthwise, then cut each half lengthwise. Cut quartered eggplant widthwise into 1/2-inch cubes. Place cubed eggplant in a perforated pan and top with salt. Refrigerate the eggplant for 30 to 40 minutes, allowing the salt to pull out the bitter liquids. When ready to cook, wipe off and discard any excess salt.

Heat 1 tablespoon of oil in a skillet on medium heat and fry shallot until golden brown. Remove shallot from oil and drain on paper towel; reserve to use as garnish.

In a frying pan, preheat 4 cups of oil. In a small mixing bowl, lightly dredge the cubed tofu with the starch. Fry tofu until crispy, then drain and reserve on paper towels until ready to use.

For the sauce: In a small sauce pan, add the sake, reduce to a quarter of the original amount. Add the remaining ingredients and whisk together thoroughly. Bring sauce to a boil, then reduce to a simmer for approximately 15 minutes.

Place a medium sauté pan over medium-high heat. Add last 2 tablespoons oil. Add cubed eggplant and sauté for 5 to 6 minutes. Add garlic and chili pepper, sauté for an additional 2 minutes, being careful not to brown the garlic. Add the reserved crispy tofu, basil, mint, and 4 ounces of sauce (or enough to coat the eggplant). Sauté eggplant for an additional minute. Place miso-glazed eggplant in the center of the dish. Top with shallots and cilantro, and serve immediately. Additional sauce can be served on the side, if desired.

Per serving (1/3 of recipe): 416 calories · 20 g fat · 2 g saturated fat · 43% calories from fat · 0 mg cholesterol · 7 g protein · 33 g carbohydrate · 11 g sugar · 4 g fiber · 3631 mg sodium · 97 mg calcium · 2 mg iron · 13 mg vitamin C · 291 mcg beta-carotene · 3 mg vitamin E

GOLDEN BEET RAVIOLI

Escopazzo, Miami, Florida

MAKES 24 RAVIOLIS (4 SERVINGS)

*E*scopazzo's name means "I am going crazy," and that pretty much sums up life in its South Beach neighborhood. But among restaurant aficionados, Escopazzo means phenomenally healthy and truly creative cuisine.

2 medium golden beets	1/2 teaspoon Celtic sea salt
1 cup Cashew 'Cheese' (recipe below)	1/2 teaspoon black pepper
juice of 1 lemon	2 cups baby arugula
1/2 cup olive oil	2 tablespoons chopped hazelnuts or
1 teaspoon white truffle-infused oil	walnuts, toasted
1 tablespoon agave nectar	

Wash the golden beets and slice them as thin as possible. If you have a slicer or mandoline, this is preferable.

Take a slice of golden beet, place a nickel-size bit of cashew cheese in the center. Close the ravioli with another slice of beet.

For the truffle-agave dressing, emulsify the lemon juice, olive oil, truffle oil, and agave nectar in a bowl. Add salt and black pepper.

Place your ravioli on a plate. Dress the arugula with the truffle-agave dressing. Place the arugula salad on top of the ravioli. Sprinkle the nuts and pour the remainder of the dressing over the beets.

CASHEW 'CHEESE'
MAKES 3 1/2 CUPS

2 cups raw cashews	1/2 teaspoon salt
water	1/2 teaspoon black pepper

Soak cashews in water for at least 5 hours. Rinse the nuts and process in a blender at high speed with salt and black pepper. Add a bit of water, but just enough to create a smooth paste.

Per serving (1/4 of recipe): 411 calories · 39 g fat · 6 g saturated fat · 82% calories from fat · 0 mg cholesterol · 5 g protein · 15 g carbohydrate · 8 g sugar · 2 g fiber · 414 mg sodium · 37 mg calcium · 2 mg iron · 7 mg vitamin C · 152 mcg beta-carotene · 5 mg vitamin E

GARLIC AND TRUFFLE WHITE BEAN DIP

Landhuis Misje, Westpunt, Curaçao

MAKES 1 1/2 CUPS

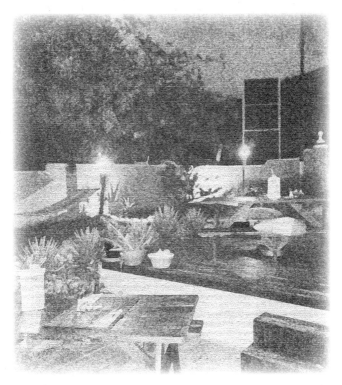

If you happen to be in beautiful Westpunt, Curaçao, make sure to stop by Landhuis Misje for dinner. Call ahead to have Anton whip up one of his delicious vegan creations for you. This dip is always on the menu.

1 15-ounce can white beans, drained
2 tablespoons lime juice
1/4 cup olive oil

1/2 teaspoon truffle oil
2 garlic cloves

Put everything in a food processor or blender. Eat with pita bread or cut up veggies.

Per serving (1/2 cup): 305 calories · 19 g fat · 3 g saturated fat · 55% calories from fat · 0 mg cholesterol · 10 g protein · 26 g carbohydrate · 1 g sugar · 6 g fiber · 299 mg sodium · 92 mg calcium · 4 mg iron · 1 mg vitamin C · 1 mcg beta-carotene · 4 mg vitamin E

MARINATED SEITAN WITH GERMAN POTATO SALAD AND OVEN-BAKED ZUCCHINI

Kopps, Berlin, Germany

MAKES 4 SERVINGS

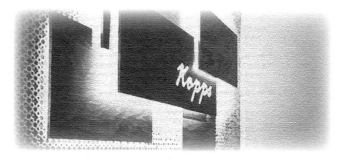

*K*opps in Berlin serves traditional German food made vegan under the watchful eye of chef Bjoern Moschinski.

POTATO SALAD

2 pounds potatoes	1/4 bunch chives, finely chopped
1/2 cup chopped onions	3/4 cup chopped gherkins
1 tablespoon olive oil	salt, to taste
1 cup vegan mayonnaise	black pepper, to taste
2 tablespoons vegetable broth	
1 tablespoon prepared mustard	

ZUCCHINI

1/4 cup olive oil	1 teaspoon dried thyme
1 garlic clove	salt, to taste
2 zucchini	lemon pepper, to taste

SEITAN

8 ounces seitan	1/2 teaspoon dried rosemary
4–6 tablespoons vegetable broth	salt, to taste
1 1/2 teaspoons garlic powder	black pepper, to taste
1 tablespoon paprika	1/4 cup olive oil
1 teaspoon dried thyme	

Ideally, prepare the potato salad a day ahead.

Boil the potatoes in salted water until tender. Rinse with cold water, peel, and cut into medium-sized cubes. Transfer to a big bowl.

Heat the oil and lightly fry the onions until translucent. Add to the potatoes.

Mix the vegan mayonnaise with vegetable broth, mustard, and chives. Pour over the potato mixture and mix thoroughly. Add gherkins. Season generously with salt and black pepper, to taste. Let cool in the fridge, preferably overnight.

The next day, taste again and season with more broth, salt, and black pepper, if necessary.

For the baked zucchini, heat the oil in a frying pan. Peel the garlic, slightly crush it with a large knife and fry in the hot oil until the clove starts to brown. Remove the clove from the oil and set the pan aside. Preheat the oven to 350°F. Rinse and thinly slice the zucchini lengthwise. Mix the garlic oil with thyme, salt, and lemon pepper. Brush the zucchini slices with the spiced oil and bake in the oven on a baking tray for about 7 minutes.

Marinate the seitan in vegetable broth with garlic powder, paprika, thyme, rosemary, salt, and black pepper.

In a hot frying pan, pan-fry the marinated seitan in oil until golden brown. Remove excess oil with paper towels, if desired.

On a plate, arrange the seitan with the cold potato salad and the baked zucchini slices.

Per serving (1/4 of recipe): 714 calories · 46 g fat · 6 g saturated fat · 57% calories from fat · 0 mg cholesterol · 21 g protein · 46 g carbohydrate · 14 g sugar · 9 g fiber · 1759 mg sodium · 153 mg calcium · 7 mg iron · 41 mg vitamin C · 1193 mcg beta-carotene · 8 mg vitamin E

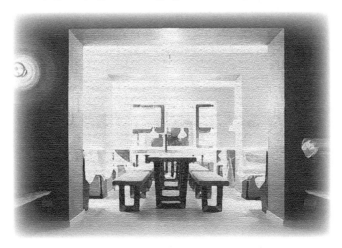

PAN-FRIED SHIITAKE

Pan Dei, Saint-Tropez, France

MAKES 4 SERVINGS

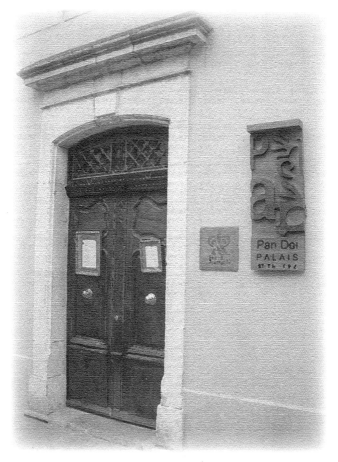

In the heart of Saint-Tropez, where partying can easily go to excess, Pan Dei is a haven of quiet beauty. Chef Renaud Capelle offers diners the very best of the Cote d'Azur.

2 cups cherry tomatoes, halved
1 tablespoon olive oil, divided
salt, to taste

black pepper, to taste
1 garlic clove, quartered
8 ounces shiitake mushrooms, sliced

Preheat the oven to 175°F.

Seed the tomato halves, using a small spoon. In a bowl, mix the tomatoes with 1/2 tablespoon olive oil, salt, black pepper, and garlic. Spread tomatoes, curved sides down, in an oven-safe dish. Cook for 20 to 25 minutes.

While tomatoes are cooking, pan-fry shiitakes in remaining 1/2 tablespoon of olive oil over medium-high heat for 4 minutes, leaving some of the mushrooms to crisp up in the pan.

Remove tomatoes from oven and mix with shiitakes.

Serve warm over pasta or rice or chilled in a salad.

Per serving (1/4 of recipe): 67 calories · 5 g fat · 0.5 g saturated fat · 51% calories from fat · 0 mg cholesterol · 2 g protein · 8 g carbohydrate · 4 g sugar · 3 g fiber · 157 mg sodium · 12 mg calcium · 0.5 mg iron · 13 mg vitamin C · 405 mcg beta-carotene · 1 mg vitamin E

Pan-Fried Tofu with Ginger and Lemongrass

Pan Dei, Saint-Tropez, France

MAKES 2 SERVINGS

4 ounces organic soft tofu
1 tablespoon olive oil
1 tablespoon sesame oil
1 bunch green onions, chopped

1 bunch fresh cilantro, chopped
1 stalk lemongrass, chopped
1-inch piece fresh ginger, chopped
3 tablespoons soy sauce

Over low heat, pan-fry the tofu in olive oil until browned, then turn, add sesame oil, and brown the second side. Add onions, cilantro, lemongrass, and ginger. Pour in the soy sauce and stir briefly to allow it to pick up the cooking juices, and then turn off the flame. Slice and serve.

Per serving (1/2 of recipe): 197 calories · 16 g fat · 2 g saturated fat · 71% calories from fat · 0 mg cholesterol · 7 g protein · 10 g carbohydrate · 3 g sugar · 2 g fiber · 1365 mg sodium · 112 mg calcium · 2 mg iron · 10 mg vitamin C · 593 mcg beta-carotene · 2 mg vitamin E

Soups

ZUPPA DI VERDURA (ITALIAN VEGETABLE SOUP)
Faraglioni, Capri, Italy

MAKES 10 SERVINGS

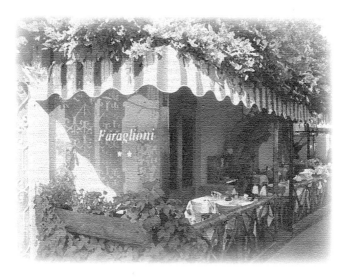

*T*he island of Capri is a quick ferry ride from the coast of Italy. A long climb up the rugged hillside leads to ancient ruins—yes, you can still see a villa built by Tiberius in classical Roman times—as well as the most modern luxuries. Faraglioni is a favorite.

3 carrots, chopped
2 cups chopped potatoes (look for interesting/unusual varieties such as purple potatoes)
1 1/2 cups chopped summer squash or zucchini
1/2 cup chopped celery
1 cup chopped green beans
1 cup green peas

1 cup chopped onion
1 tablespoon water ~~or olive~~ oil
6 cups water or vegetable broth (enough to cover the vegetables)
salt, to taste
black pepper, to taste
handful of fresh herbs such as basil, oregano, rosemary, and/or parsley (optional)

Sauté vegetables in a small amount of water or olive oil for about five minutes. This step can be skipped if preferred, or if you're short on time.

Add enough water or vegetable broth to just cover the vegetables (approximately 6 cups). Add a touch of salt and black pepper and bring soup to a boil. Stir in fresh herbs, if using. Upon boiling, reduce to a simmer and cook until vegetables are tender, but still firm and colorful. Be careful not to overcook the soup.

Serve hot and then refrigerate/reheat leftovers as desired.

Per serving, (1/10 of recipe): 52 calories · 0.2 g fat · 0 g saturated fat · 3% calories from fat · 0 mg cholesterol · 2 g protein · 12 g carbohydrate · 3 g sugar · 3 g fiber · 179 mg sodium · 34 mg calcium · 1 mg iron · 8 mg vitamin C · 1635 mcg beta-carotene · 0.2 mg vitamin E

WHITE GAZPACHO
Elizabeth's Gone Raw, Washington, District of Columbia

MAKES 4 SERVINGS

*E*lizabeth takes raw foods to a whole new level in her classically beautiful restaurant.

WHITE GAZPACHO

4 cucumbers, peeled	1 head celery
3 pounds parsnips, peeled	1 quart chamomile almond milk, recipe
2 cups cashews (soaked for a minimum	below
of two hours and then drained)	lemon juice, to taste (optional)
3 pounds green seedless grapes	salt, to taste

CHAMOMILE ALMOND MILK

2 cups soaked almonds	6 bags chamomile, emptied
2 quarts water	

Blend almonds and water; pass through a nut milk bag. Place almond milk back into blender with chamomile and blend for 20 seconds. Pour into container and let rest overnight, strain next day.

Juice all fruits and vegetables, then add in Chamomile Almond Milk and place into a blender with cashews, blend and pass through a nut milk bag. Adjust with salt and lemon juice if needed.

Per serving (1/4 of recipe): 775 calories · 47 g fat · 7 g saturated fat · 50% calories from fat · 0 mg cholesterol · 22 g protein · 78 g carbohydrate · 52 g sugar · 10 g fiber · 589 mg sodium · 220 mg calcium · 7 mg iron · 5 mg vitamin C · 427 mcg beta-carotene · 10 mg vitamin E

CALIFORNIA GOLD CHILI

Chili Addiction, Hollywood, California

MAKES 5 SERVINGS

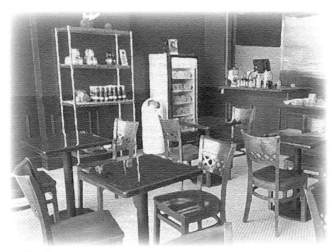

*Y*es, it really is habit-forming.

1 Spanish onion, chopped
3 garlic cloves, minced
1 red bell pepper, chopped
2 tablespoons olive oil
2 pounds firm organic tofu, drained
1 15-ounce can diced tomatoes
1 15-ounce can pinto beans, drained
1 jalapeno pepper, seeds removed, minced

2 tablespoons dried ground California chilies
2 tablespoons ground ancho chili powder
1 tablespoon dry vegetable soup mix
1 teaspoon dried cumin
1 1/2 cups water
salt, to taste

Sauté onion, garlic, and bell pepper in olive oil until browned, then crumble in drained tofu by hand.

Add all remaining ingredients to the pot and bring to a boil.

After bringing to a boil, turn down to a low simmer and cook for an hour. You may need to add more water to achieve the perfect consistency.

Per serving (1/5 of recipe): 309 calories · 14 g fat · 3 g saturated fat · 40% calories from fat · 0 mg cholesterol · 22 g protein · 29 g carbohydrate · 6 g sugar · 10 g fiber · 462 mg sodium · 441 mg calcium · 6 mg iron · 54 mg vitamin C · 1384 mcg beta-carotene · 4 mg vitamin E

INDIAN PAPAYA SOUP

Hotel Capitan Suizo, Guanacaste, Costa Rica

MAKES 2 SERVINGS

The village of Tamarindo is known for its perfect surf and sandy beaches, and there is a delightful touch of Switzerland in the Hotel Capitán Suizo. It is a perfectly kept hotel that rolls out the red carpet for the howler monkeys, parrots, and urracas who pass by, as well as the orphaned animals that the locals often bring here. The menu is kind, too, with many delicious, plant-based dishes.

1 medium onion, chopped	1/2 teaspoon dried coriander seeds
2 garlic cloves, chopped	8 cloves
2 tablespoons sunflower oil *broth*	3/4 teaspoon salt *Table Taste*
1 medium papaya, chopped	1 1/4 cups vegetable broth
1 pinch powdered ginger	1 pinch white pepper
1 pinch ground cumin	1 pinch curry powder

Sauté the onion and garlic in the sunflower oil *broth*, then add all remaining ingredients and cook until the papaya is tender, about 15 minutes. Remove the cloves. Place the mixture in a blender or food processor on the lowest speed and blend until smooth. Serve immediately.

Per serving (1/2 of recipe): 221 calories · 14 g fat · 2 g saturated fat · 57% calories from fat · 0 mg cholesterol · 2 g protein · 25 g carbohydrate · 16 g sugar · 4 g fiber · 1486 mg sodium · 56 mg calcium · 1 mg iron · 96 mg vitamin C · 571 mcg beta-carotene · 6 mg vitamin E

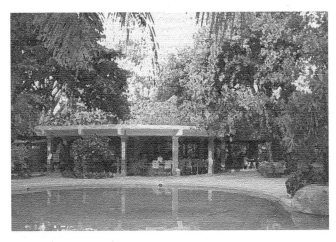

MELON SOUP WITH PROSECCO

3/4 C. Wine

La Tomate, Washington, District of Columbia

SERVES 10

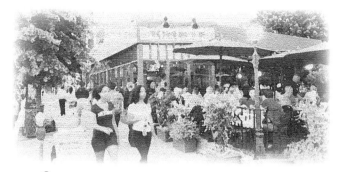

$\mathcal{J}$ust off Dupong Circle, one of Washington, D.C.'s busiest neighborhoods, La Tomate is an oasis of delicious foods. This soup is a delight for the eyes and taste buds.

1 honeydew melon	1/4 cup Prosecco *wine* for honeydew melon
1 cantaloupe	1/2 cup Prosecco for cantaloupe

Peel the skin of both the honey dew and cantaloupe melons. Dice in small pieces.

Mix the melons separately using a high speed blender until just about smooth, then add Prosecco at the end. Mix well but make sure the consistency is the same for both honeydew and cantaloupe.

Mix together just before serving as the fiber and water content will separate. Add more Prosecco if desired.

Per serving (1/10 of recipe): 79 calories · 0.3 g fat · 0 g saturated fat · 3% calories from fat · 0 mg cholesterol · 1 g protein · 17 g carbohydrate · 15 g sugar · 2 g fiber · 33 mg sodium · 14 mg calcium · 0.4 mg iron · 43 mg vitamin C · 1153 mcg beta-carotene · 0 mg vitamin E

PASSATO DI VERDURE FRESCHE

Linus Bar Ristorante, Cannigione, Sardinia

MAKES 4 SERVINGS

$\mathcal{J}$n Sardinia's extreme northern end, rocky hillsides and vineyards are far more common than vegetable gardens.

Even so, Salvatore Demontes and his team deliver a delicious vegetable soup. See if you notice the subtle differences between two Italian vegetable soups, this one from Sardinia and another from Capri (page 14).

3 carrots   3 celery stalks
3 zucchini   water
1 fennel bulb   *Table*   salt, to taste
3 small potatoes   *Taste*   black pepper, to taste
1 onion

Thoroughly clean vegetables, scrubbing the skins to remove hidden bits of soil. Cut vegetables into roughly 2 to 3-inch pieces. Place in a pot and cover with water. Bring to a boil, and then reduce the temperature so that the vegetables cook at a moderate to low temperature for 30 minutes. Vegetables are done when they can be pierced easily with a fork.

Remove from heat and let cool for 5 minutes. Using an immersion blender, blend vegetables in the pot until smooth. You can also use a blender, making sure that soup is cooled and is blended in small batches. Heat to desired temperature and season with salt and black pepper to taste. Can be served hot, chilled, or at room temperature.

Per serving (1/4 of recipe): 158 calories · 1 g fat · 0.2 g saturated fat · 5 % calories from fat · 0 mg cholesterol · 5 g protein · 36 g carbohydrate · 10 g sugar · 8 g fiber · 248 mg sodium · 113 mg calcium · 3 mg iron · 42 mg vitamin C · 4478 mcg beta-carotene · 1 mg vitamin E

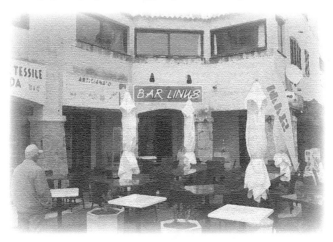

WHITE BEAN BISQUE WITH TOFU MOUSSE, RADISH RELISH, AND CRISPY SHALLOTS

Ashby Inn, Paris, Virginia

MAKES 8 SERVINGS

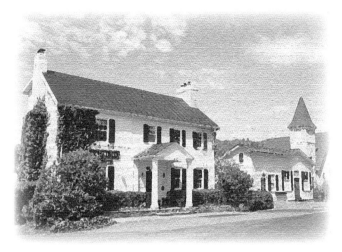

*I*n rural Virginia, delicious flavors and culinary creativity at the Ashby Inn make time seem to stand still.

3 quarts water
2 cups dried white navy beans (soaked overnight in water, discard floating skins)
3 garlic cloves, minced

2 shallots, minced
1 tablespoon olive oil
sea salt, to taste
black pepper, to taste

Bring the water to a simmer with the beans, garlic, and shallots. Cover and cook for 45 to 50 minutes, or until the beans are completely tender.

In a high-powered food processor, blend the cooked beans and their liquid in batches until the mixture is completely smooth.

Drizzle in some of the olive oil. Season with salt and black pepper and repeat until the olive oil is incorporated. Check seasoning and adjust as necessary with salt.

Transfer the soup back to the pot and reheat the soup until hot, but not boiling.

Serve in individual bowls, with a tablespoon of the tofu mousse (recipe below) and a tablespoon of the radish relish (recipe below).

Hide the tofu and relish with a sprinkle of crispy shallots (recipe below).

Add more of the shallots to the soup at the last possible moment, so the shallots retain their crunchiness.

TOFU MOUSSE (MAKES ABOUT 1 CUP)

8 ounces firm silken tofu   3/4 teaspoon salt
2 garlic cloves

Blend tofu and garlic until smooth in a food processor. Season with salt and keep cold.

RADISH RELISH (MAKES ABOUT 4 CUPS)

5 cups black radishes (cut in tiny squares)   3 cups julienned red radish
1 cup sugar   1 bunch chives, chopped
1 cup red wine vinegar   1/4 cup virgin olive oil
    1/4 teaspoon salt, or to taste

Cook the black radish with the sugar and vinegar until thick and "jammy," about 15 minutes, stirring regularly.

Let mixture cool. Mix in the rest of the ingredients. Salt to taste.

FRIED SHALLOTS (MAKES ABOUT 3/4 CUP)

5 large shallots   1 quart peanut oil
1 cup rice flour

Shave the shallots as thinly as possible, and soak them in ice water for one hour.

Heat the oil in a deep sided pot to 325°F.

Drain the shallots and shake dry. Toss the shallots in the rice flour. Shake off the excess flour and fry in batches until golden brown.

Drain the shallots on paper towels.

Per serving (1/8 of recipe): 283 calories · 4 g fat · 1 g saturated fat · 14% calories from fat · 0 mg cholesterol · 12 g protein · 50 g carbohydrate · 5 g sugar · 14 g fiber · 293 mg sodium · 114 mg calcium · 3 mg iron · 6 mg vitamin C · 53 mcg beta-carotene · 0.5 mg vitamin E

CUCUMBER GAZPACHO

Hotel Capitán Suizo, Guanacaste, Costa Rica

MAKES 5 SERVINGS

3 cups cucumber (peeled and cut into chunks)
1 garlic clove
1/2 cup non-dairy creamer

1/2 cup plain non-dairy yogurt
2/3 cup ice
salt, to taste
fresh basil leaves, for garnish (optional)

Place all ingredients in a blender and blend until creamy. If desired, place a basil leaf on top for decoration.

Per serving (1/5 of recipe): 55 calories · 2 g fat · 0.5 g saturated fat · 37% calories from fat · 0 mg cholesterol · 1 g protein · 8 g carbohydrate · 4 g sugar · 1 g fiber · 156 mg sodium · 48 mg calcium · 0.5 mg iron · 6 mg vitamin C · 27 mcg beta-carotene · 0.2 mg vitamin E

SEA VEGETABLE CHOWDER

Six Main, Chester, Connecticut

MAKES 4 SERVINGS

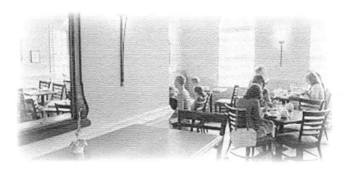

*T*his unusual vegetarian farm-to-table restaurant in Chester, Connecticut, serves the very freshest organic food.

1 handful dried seaweed (such as hijiki, arame, wakame)
6 cups vegetable broth
1/4 cup coconut oil
1/2 small onion, chopped
2 celery stalks, chopped
1/2 cup chopped mushrooms
2 carrots, chopped
2 or 3 thyme sprigs
2 garlic cloves

salt, to taste
black pepper, to taste
1/4 cup gluten-free flour, such as garbanzo flour or rice flour
2 medium potatoes, chopped
1/2 cup cashew milk (see recipe below)
red pepper flakes, to taste (optional)
Cashew Milk (makes about 2 cups):
1 cup soaked cashews
2 cups water

Blend until smooth. Strain out pulp.

Soak the sea vegetables in the vegetable broth for 15 minutes. Strain the vegetable broth for the soup and set aside the sea vegetables.

Heat the oil in a sauce pan and sauté the onion, celery, mushrooms, and carrots until the onion is translucent. Add the thyme and the garlic. Season with salt and black pepper to taste. Add the gluten-free flour and stir a minute or two until all the flour is absorbed into the oil and vegetable mixture.

Add the vegetable broth and potatoes and bring to a boil. Simmer until potatoes are cooked and begin to break down a little in the broth. Chop the soaked sea vegetables into bite-size pieces and add to the soup.

When the potatoes are cooked, stir in the cashew milk and simmer a little longer until soup begins to thicken. Add more vegetable broth if it's too thick for your taste. Throw in red pepper flakes at the end if you want a little kick.

Per serving (1/4 of recipe): 301 calories · 18 g fat · 13 g saturated fat · 51% calories from fat · 0 mg cholesterol · 5 g protein · 34 g carbohydrate · 8 g sugar · 5 g fiber · 1648 mg sodium · 67 mg calcium · 3 mg iron · 17 mg vitamin C · 2790 mcg beta-carotene · 1 mg vitamin E

MUSHROOM SOUP
Sushiko, Washington, District of Columbia

MAKES 1 SERVING

 qual parts Asian tradition and modern flavor, Sushiko serves some of the best fusion cuisine anywhere.

1 cup water
1 piece kombu
1/4 teaspoon salt
1 1/2 teaspoons soy sauce

1 ounce dried seasonal wild mushrooms (for example: enoki, chanterelle, shimeji, or blend of preferred mushrooms)

Bring to a boil, then cook on medium heat for 10 minutes and serve.

Per serving: 89 calories · 0.3 g fat · 0 g saturated fat · 3% calories from fat · 0 mg cholesterol · 3 g protein · 22 g carbohydrate · 7 g sugar · 4 g fiber · 1056 mg sodium · 14 mg calcium · 1 mg iron · 1 mg vitamin C · 95 mcg beta-carotene · 0 mg vitamin E

TOMATO BASIL SOUP

Old Dungeon Ghyll Hotel, Cumbria, England

MAKES 4 SERVINGS

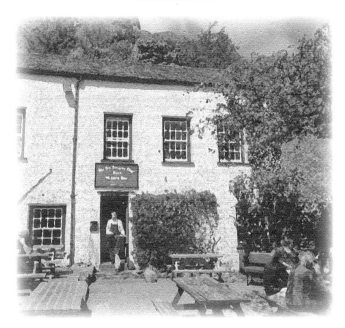

In England's Lake District, a ghyll is a narrow stream or a wooded ravine, and the Old Dungeon Ghyll Hotel is where serious hikers kick their boots off at the end of a strenuous day.

1 large onion, chopped
1/2 tablespoon caraway seeds
1 tablespoon olive oil
1 15-ounce can chopped tomatoes (Italian plum)

1 15-ounce can white beans, such as cannellini or white kidney (optional)
1/2–3/4 cup chopped fresh basil
salt, to taste
black pepper, to taste

Sauté onion and caraway seeds in olive oil until the onion is soft. Add the tomatoes, beans, if using, and basil and bring to a boil and let it cook for 5 minutes. Purée the mixture, adding more water if you like it thinner. If desired, continue to cook on the stove for 5 additional minutes. Add salt and black pepper to taste.

Per serving (1/4 cup): 66 calories · 4 g fat · 0.5 g saturated fat · 50% calories from fat · 0 mg cholesterol · 2 g protein · 8 g carbohydrate · 4 g sugar · 2 g fiber · 301 mg sodium · 56 mg calcium · 1 mg iron · 13 mg vitamin C · 243 mcg beta-carotene · 1 mg vitamin E

TOMATO-COCONUT SOUP
Kopps, Berlin, Germany

MAKES 4 SERVINGS

water
2 pounds tomatoes
5 tablespoons olive oil
2 onions, chopped
1 tablespoon sugar
1/4 cup tomato paste

17 fluid ounces vegetable broth
17 fluid ounces coconut milk
1 bunch fresh basil
salt, to taste
black pepper, to taste

Fill a pot half way with water and bring to a boil. Have a bowl with cold or ice water ready.

Remove the stems from the tomatoes and cut a cross into the bottom of each tomato. When the water is boiling, blanch the prepared tomatoes for 10 to 15 seconds, remove, and put them into the ice water.

Now you can easily peel the tomatoes. Cut the peeled tomatoes into small cubes. Set aside.

In a pot, heat the olive oil and add the onions and sugar. As soon as the onions start to brown, add the tomato paste and cook for 2 to 3 minutes. Add the chopped tomatoes and cook for 5 more minutes.

Cover with the broth and coconut milk and cook on low heat for 15 minutes.

Rinse the basil and roughly cut it. Add the basil and the soup to a blender or food processor and blend until smooth. Season with salt and black pepper to taste and serve hot.

Per serving (1/4 of recipe): 478 calories · 42 g fat · 25 g saturated fat · 76% calories from fat · 0 mg cholesterol · 5 g protein · 26 g carbohydrate · 18 g sugar · 5 g fiber · 811 mg sodium · 61 mg calcium · 3 mg iron · 46 mg vitamin C · 1082 mcg beta-carotene · 4 mg vitamin E

Salads

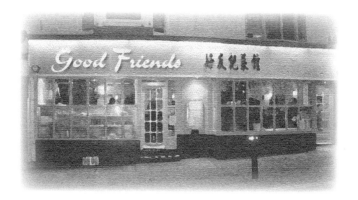

CHINESE GREENS
Good Friends, Brighton, England

Chinese greens are delicious, healthful, and easy to prepare, but are virtually unknown to Westerners. In fact, Chinese restaurants in Western countries often leave them off their English-language menus. At Good Friends restaurant in Brighton, England, the staff is glad to interpret Chinese traditions for western tastes.

Here are the vegetables, with their Cantonese names:

Tong choi (冬菜) or morning glory (sometimes called Chinese water spinach), is a delicious and mild-flavored green, with thin hollow stalks and soft leaves, both of which are eaten. Tong choi means "hollow vegetable."

Bok choi (白菜), whose name means "white vegetable," is among the most familiar vegetables, with fat stalks and mild flavor.

Choi sum (菜心) means "vegetable heart."

Gai-lan, or *kai-lan* (芥蘭), is Chinese broccoli. Its name means "mustard orchid," hinting at its slightly bitter flavor.

Dau myoo (豆苗) or mange-tout shoots (or pea pod tips), are the tender shoots from the plant that also produces the better-known mange-tout pods.

Si yong choi (西洋菜) is watercress. Its name means "vegetable from the west ocean." It is used mainly in soups, but can be sautéed or cooked in other ways, and also served raw.

Fang shu myoo (紅薯苗) is a sweet potato shoot.

Bo choi (菠菜) is spinach.

Lan gua myoo (南瓜苗) is pumpkin shoot.

The usual method for preparing greens is very quick. Simply heat a small amount of oil in a wok, and then add crushed or minced garlic. Then add salt, followed by the greens. Stir occasionally. When the greens are soft and have collapsed to a fraction of their raw bulk, they are ready to serve.

WARM SPINACH SALAD
Sushiko, Washington, District of Columbia

MAKES 2 SERVINGS

4 cups fresh baby spinach
1/4 cup shredded carrots

2 tablespoons bamboo shoots
4 ounces sliced shiitake mushrooms

DRESSING

2 teaspoons sake
2 teaspoons soy sauce
2 teaspoons mirin
2 garlic cloves, chopped

2 teaspoons black bean sauce
2 teaspoons canola oil
1 teaspoon fresh grated ginger

Toss the baby spinach, shredded carrots, and bamboo shoots in a serving bowl.

Sauté ingredients for dressing on medium heat in a small saucepan for 3 minutes, stirring constantly. During the last minute, add the sliced mushrooms and continue stirring. Once finished, pour the dressing mixture over the spinach mixture. Toss and serve.

Per serving (1/2 of recipe): 109 calories · 5 g fat · 0.5 g saturated fat · 42% calories from fat · 0 mg cholesterol · 4 g protein · 11 g carbohydrate · 4 g sugar · 3 g fiber · 479 mg sodium · 74 mg calcium · 2 mg iron · 19 mg vitamin C · 4516 mcg beta-carotene · 2 mg vitamin E

POLENTA AND ORANGE SALAD
Plum Bistro, Seattle, Washington

*I*n a word, wow! There is a reason the place is always packed, and you'll discover it as soon as the server presents your plate.

MAKES 4 SERVINGS

6 cups arugula
2 cups Fennel Salsa (recipe follows)

1/4 cup Cilantro-Orange Vinaigrette (recipe follows)
8 Polenta Cakes (recipe follows)

In a large bowl, combine arugula and fennel salsa. Dress the combined arugula and salsa mixture with cilantro-orange vinaigrette.

Divide between four plates and arrange two polenta cakes by the side of the greens on each plate.

FENNEL SALSA
MAKES 2 CUPS

1 tablespoon olive oil
2 tablespoons white wine vinegar
2 tablespoons roughly chopped fresh cilantro
2 teaspoons gluten-free tamari
2 teaspoons minced fresh ginger
2 teaspoons sugar
3 medium oranges, peeled, segmented, and pith and membranes removed

(it's okay to use a variety of oranges here, such as blood orange, navels, or any other type readily available)
1 medium fennel bulb, trimmed and sliced in julienne strips
1/2 cup thinly sliced red onion
sea salt, to taste
freshly ground black pepper, to taste

In a medium bowl, mix together oil, vinegar, cilantro, tamari, ginger, and sugar. Gently stir in orange segments, fennel, and onion. Season with sea salt and freshly ground black pepper.

CILANTRO-ORANGE VINAIGRETTE
MAKES 10 TABLESPOONS

1 tablespoon white wine vinegar
1 tablespoon finely minced fresh cilantro
1 tablespoon soy sauce
1 tablespoon chopped fresh ginger

1 teaspoon maple syrup
1 teaspoon sugar
2 tablespoons olive oil
1/4 cup orange juice, preferably fresh-squeezed

In a medium bowl, whisk together vinegar, cilantro, soy sauce, ginger, maple syrup, sugar, olive oil, and orange juice. Set aside.

· POLENTA CAKES
MAKES 8 CAKES

3 cups water
1/4 teaspoon sea salt
1 cup cornmeal

6 tablespoons garlic-ginger oil (recipe follows)

Bring 3 cups of water and sea salt to a boil in a large sauce-pan. Add cornmeal and cook, stirring frequently, for about 10 minutes or until cornmeal thickens. Stir in garlic-ginger oil, being sure to scoop in a generous amount of the ginger and garlic pieces.

Spread polenta into a medium pan or casserole dish, such as a 9 x 9-inch Pyrex. Cover and refrigerate about 4–5 hours or overnight.

When ready to prepare the dish, cut the polenta with a 1 1/2-inch cookie cutter into 10–12 disks. (For an extra layer of flavor before reheating, spray cakes with cooking spray, heat a grill to medium heat, and cook cakes 3 to 4 minutes on each side to form grill marks.) Or you can warm the cakes by putting a medium grill pan on medium heat. Add the cakes along with 1–2 tablespoons of water, just enough to steam but not bake them. Cook for 3 minutes on each side or until warmed through.

GARLIC-GINGER OIL
MAKES 6 TABLESPOONS

2 tablespoons canola oil
2 tablespoons minced fresh garlic

2 tablespoons minced fresh ginger

In a large sauté pan, heat oil over medium-high heat. Add garlic and ginger and cook for 5 to 7 minutes, until browned. Remove from heat and allow to cool. Any oil that is not used for the recipe can be stored in the refrigerator for 2 to 3 weeks.

Per serving (1/4 of recipe): 365 calories · 14 g fat · 1 g saturated fat · 34% calories from fat · 0 mg cholesterol · 6 g protein · 56 g carbohydrate · 17 g sugar · 7 g fiber · 602 mg sodium · 139 mg calcium · 3 mg iron · 70 mg vitamin C · 608 mcg beta-carotene · 3 mg vitamin E

POIVRADE

Sénéquier, Saint-Tropez, France

MAKES 4 SERVINGS

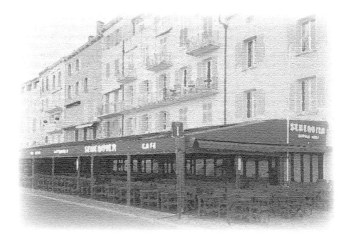

*T*his delightful starter comes from the Sénéquier—the essential place for an afternoon drink while watching yachts and passersby at the Saint-Tropez harbor.

Poivrade artichokes are small, violet-tinged, and much more flavorful than the common globe (or Camus) artichokes, with almost no choke. They are common in the south of France where this dish would typically be sprinkled with a bit of parmesan.

4 small artichokes	3/4 cup vegetable broth
juice of 1 lemon	1 garlic clove
2 tablespoons olive oil	sea salt
1 bay leaf	freshly ground black pepper
1/4 cup white wine	

Cut 1 inch from the top of the artichoke leaves, then cut leaves off with a knife or scissors until you get to the thin pale leaves underneath. Cut the stalk to about 1 inch from the bulb. Then slice the artichoke in half lengthwise. Sprinkle with some of the lemon juice to prevent discoloration.

In a saucepan, heat the olive oil and bay leaf, then add the artichokes, cut side up. Add the wine, broth, remaining lemon juice, and garlic, and cook uncovered over low heat for about 15 minutes or until cooked thoroughly, adding more broth if the liquid evaporates. Cool in the refrigerator for an hour.

Place the artichokes in a shallow bowl, and season with salt and black pepper.

Per serving (1/4 of recipe): 130 calories · 7 g fat · 1 g saturated fat · 48 % calories from fat · 0 mg cholesterol · 3 g protein · 14 g carbohydrate · 2 g sugar · 9 g fiber · 385 mg sodium · 26 mg calcium · 1 mg iron · 11 mg vitamin C · 54 mcg beta-carotene · 1 mg vitamin E

HEIRLOOM TOMATO SALAD

Elizabeth's Gone Raw, Washington, District of Columbia

MAKES 4 SERVINGS

3 heirloom tomatoes, cut into bite-size pieces
1 tablespoon walnut oil
salt, to taste
black pepper, to taste

juice of 1/2 lemon
2 fennel bulbs, cored and thinly sliced
1 teaspoon fresh marjoram leaves
2 tablespoons Shallot Hemp Milk Vinaigrette (recipe below)

Toss tomatoes with walnut oil, salt, and black pepper. Add in half of the lemon juice, taste, and re-season if necessary.

In a separate bowl, place fennel, remaining lemon juice, salt, and black pepper, then tear by hand the marjoram leaves and toss together. Re-season if needed.

To plate, place dressing on the bottom of a bowl, arrange the tomatoes in small groups, and top with the fennel salad.

SHALLOT HEMP MILK VINAIGRETTE
MAKES ABOUT 5 1/2 CUPS

1 1/2 cups cashews (soaked in water for a few hours, then drained)
1 cup hemp seeds
3 cups water

1 tablespoon dry mustard
1 tablespoon chopped shallots
salt, to taste
white pepper, to taste

Blend all ingredients together, and season to taste with salt and white pepper.

Per serving (1/4 of recipe): 129 calories · 7 g fat · 1 g saturated fat · 48% calories from fat · 0 mg cholesterol · 4 g protein · 15 g carbohydrate · 7 g sugar · 6 g fiber · 268 mg sodium · 78 mg calcium · 2 mg iron · 28 mg vitamin C · 571 mcg beta-carotene · 1 mg vitamin E

HEART OF LETTUCE WITH FRENCH GREEN BEANS

Sénéquier, Saint-Tropez, France

MAKES 2 SERVINGS

1/2 cup French green beans
2 teaspoons olive oil
1 teaspoon lemon juice

Sea salt, to taste
Freshly ground black pepper, to taste
1 head butter (Boston) lettuce

Cook the green beans in salted boiling water and then chill in ice water. Whisk together oil, lemon juice, salt, and pepper. Wash the lettuce and remove any rough outer leaves. Cut the lettuce head in half and place in two shallow bowls, top with green beans, drizzling the dressing over the salad.

Per serving (1/2 of recipe): 60 calories · 5 g fat · 1 g saturated fat · 69% calories from fat · 0 mg cholesterol · 2 g protein · 4 g carbohydrate · 1 g sugar · 2 g fiber · 230 mg sodium · 41 mg calcium · 1 mg iron · 6 mg vitamin C · 1730 mcg beta-carotene · 1 mg vitamin E

Main Dishes

FETTUCCINE TARTUFO E FUNGHI
Smeraldo, Rome, Italy

MAKES 6 SERVINGS

*A*mong the countless streetside restaurants in Rome waiting to pour wine and serve pizza to tourists, dating couples, and anyone else who passes by, Smeraldo stands out. Its friendly atmosphere and delicious food set the stage for a perfect evening.

TRUFFLE CREAM SAUCE (MAKES 2 CUPS)

1 tablespoon olive oil	salt, to taste (optional)
1 tablespoon whole-wheat flour	4 garlic cloves
2 cups unsweetened non-dairy milk	8 ounces white mushrooms, sliced
1/2 cup raw cashews	2 tablespoons dried oregano
1 tablespoon nutritional yeast	14 ounces dry fettuccine
1 tablespoon truffle oil	salt, to taste

Sauce: Place a saucepan over medium heat. Add the oil, then add the flour. Whisk constantly as flour cooks, about 3 minutes. Add the non-dairy milk and lower the heat. Simmer, whisking often, until the sauce reaches the desired consistency. (Usually this takes about 15 minutes.) Process cashews in a food processor until they are very fine. Pour the sauce, nutritional yeast, and truffle oil into the cashews and blend. Season with salt if desired.

Pasta: Mince the garlic and cook over low heat in frying pan. Add the mushrooms and cook until tender. Add the truffle cream sauce and oregano to the mushrooms. Meanwhile cook the pasta according to package directions until al dente. Once the pasta is ready, mix the pasta and sauce together in the pan.

Per serving (1/6 of recipe): 419 calories · 12 g fat · 2 g saturated fat · 25% calories from fat · 0 mg cholesterol · 16 g protein · 62 g carbohydrate · 3 g sugar · 6 g fiber · 180 mg sodium · 139 mg calcium · 4 mg iron · 2 mg vitamin C · 11 mcg beta-carotene · 1 mg vitamin E

DAAL BAATI
Imperial Palace, Rajkot, Gujarat, India

In the state of Gujarat in western India, Rajkot is off the beaten path for most Westerners. But the Imperial Palace offers some of the most savory dishes anywhere.

It is important that Baati be removed from the oven immediately after it is done. Otherwise, if left in the oven for a longer time, Baati may turn hard.

DAAL
MAKES 5 SERVINGS

1/3 cup toor daal (yellow pigeon peas)	2 medium tomatoes, chopped
1/3 cup yellow mung daal	2 tablespoons vegan margarine
1/4 cup masoor daal (red split lentils)	2 teaspoons cumin seeds
1/4 cup chana daal (split bengal gram)	2 teaspoons coriander seeds
4 cups water	2 teaspoons mustard seeds
salt, to taste	2 teaspoons fennel seeds
1 teaspoon turmeric powder	1/2 teaspoon asafetida
1 teaspoon chopped ginger	1/4 cup chopped onion
1 teaspoon chopped garlic	1 1/2 teaspoons red chili powder
1 fresh green chili, chopped	coriander leaves (optional)

Wash the daal and soak in water for 30 minutes, then drain. Put the daal in a pan, add 4 cups water, salt, turmeric, ginger, garlic, green chili, and tomatoes. Bring to a boil, then cook for 20 minutes over low heat.

Heat margarine in a wok, add cumin, coriander, mustard, fennel seeds, and asafetida. When the seeds start to crackle, add chopped onion and keep stirring. When the onion becomes light brown, add chili powder and then immediately put this mixture into the boiled daal. Boil it for another 5 minutes.

Garnish with coriander leaves, if using.

BAATI
MAKES 20 PEDHA

3 cups whole-wheat flour, divided	1/2 teaspoon baking powder
1 cup semolina	3 tablespoons vegan margarine
1 teaspoon salt	water

Preheat oven to 390°F. Mix 2 1/2 cups whole-wheat flour, semolina, salt, baking powder, and vegan margarine. Knead the mixture and add water as needed to form dough. Cover with a moist cloth and let sit for 20 minutes. Divide dough into 20 portions, flattening into circles to make "pedha." Dust baking tray with remaining 1/2 cup flour and arrange pedha for baking. Bake for 20 to 30 minutes.

Per serving (1/5 of daal recipe plus 5 pedha): 625 calories · 14 g fat · 3 g saturated fat · 19% calories from fat · 0 mg cholesterol · 25 g protein · 107 g carbohydrate · 4 g sugar · 21 g fiber · 795 mg sodium · 122 mg calcium · 8 mg iron · 30 mg vitamin C · 394 mcg beta-carotene · 2 mg vitamin E

LIVING VEGETABLE LASAGNETTA

Escopazzo, Miami, Florida

MAKES 8 SERVINGS

1 cup extra-virgin olive oil	1 cup grated zucchini
juice of 1 lemon	1 cup grated eggplant
4 or 5 basil leaves, chopped	1 cup grated butternut squash
sea salt, to taste	1 cup grated fennel
black pepper, to taste	Chive and Dill Cashew Cheese (recipe
1 cup grated carrots	follows)

Whisk together olive oil, lemon juice, basil, salt, and black pepper. Place the grated vegetables in individual bowls, and divide the dressing among the 5 vegetables, mixing to coat fully.

Assemble the lasagna in an 8 x 8-inch pan, alternating layers of vegetables (one type per layer) and cashew cheese. Refrigerate for 3 to 5 hours, allowing it to set.

CHIVE AND DILL CASHEW CHEESE

2 cups raw cashews	salt, to taste
1/3–1/2 cup chopped chives	black pepper, to taste
3 tablespoons chopped fresh dill	1 tablespoon apple cider vinegar

Soak cashews in water for 5 hours. Rinse cashews and drain, process in a blender at high speed with chives and dill. Season with salt and black pepper. Add apple cider vinegar.

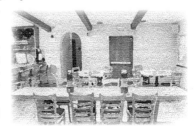

Per serving (1/8 of recipe): 439 calories · 41 g fat · 6 g saturated fat · 82% calories from fat · 0 mg cholesterol · 7 g protein · 15 g carbohydrate · 4 g sugar · 3 g fiber · 317 mg sodium · 36 mg calcium · 3 mg iron · 10 mg vitamin C · 1928 mcg beta-carotene · 5 mg vitamin E

CANELONES DE VERDURAS
Krystal Restaurant, Tenerife, Spain

MAKES 3 SERVINGS

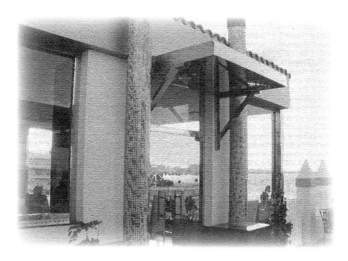

$\mathcal{T}$he Krystal Restaurant perches on the balcony of the Riu Palace hotel overlooking the black volcanic beach of the island of Tenerife, a Spanish island off the coast of Africa. The clientele, having fled the winters of Germany, Belgium, Holland, and Britain, dine on elegant fare.

SAUCE
1 pound mushrooms, sliced
1/4 cup water
1/4 cup white wine, sherry, or vegetable broth
1 1/2 cups unsweetened soymilk
2 tablespoons vegan margarine

1/4 cup nutritional yeast (optional, if using, increase water by 1/4 cup)
1 teaspoon balsamic vinegar
salt, to taste
black pepper, to taste

PASTA
12 dried cannelloni noodles (if cannelloni is unavailable use lasagna noodles)

FILLING
2 tablespoons vegan margarine
1 large or 2 small zucchini, peeled and chopped into small cubes
3 large or 4 small carrots, peeled and chopped into small cubes

1/2 pound asparagus, sliced into 1/4-inch pieces
4 garlic cloves, chopped
1 teaspoon dried tarragon
1 teaspoon dried thyme

36

| 1/2 cup unsweetened soymilk | salt, to taste |
| 1/4 cup flour | black pepper, to taste |

For the sauce: In a large skillet or wok, cook the mushrooms uncovered in 1/4 cup water plus 1/4 cup white wine, sherry, or vegetable broth on medium heat with occasional stirring for 15 minutes, or until the water is mostly evaporated. Add 1 1/2 cups soymilk and 2 tablespoons vegan margarine and stir gently. Turn heat to low, cover, and simmer 25 minutes.

When the mushrooms are done, transfer to blender. Add 1/4 cup nutritional yeast (if using) and 1 teaspoon balsamic vinegar and blend well. Transfer mushroom sauce to a microwavable bowl or 2-quart saucepan. Add salt and black pepper to taste. Set aside. (Note: The mushroom sauce can be made in advance and stored chilled.)

For the pasta: Cook the cannelloni noodles according to package directions. When the pasta is done, pour off boiling water and arrange the noodles on a plate so they will not stick together as they cool.

For the filling: Melt 2 tablespoons vegan margarine in a large non-stick skillet on medium-high heat (you can use the same skillet you used for the mushrooms). Add the zucchini, carrots, asparagus, and garlic and cook with occasional stirring until vegetables are tender, about 5 to 10 minutes.

Add the tarragon, thyme, 1/2 cup soymilk, and 1/4 cup of flour. Stir well to combine. Turn heat to low and cook for 10 minutes with occasional stirring. Add salt and black pepper to taste.

Stuff the cooked cannelloni with the vegetable mixture. If using lasagna noodles place 2 tablespoons of vegetables on top of each noodle and roll it into a short tube.

If needed, re-heat the mushroom sauce in the microwave or on low heat on the stovetop. Spoon the mushroom sauce onto the pasta and serve.

Per serving (1/3 of recipe): 593 calories · 18 g fat · 4 g saturated fat · 26% calories from fat · 0 mg cholesterol · 22 g protein · 87 g carbohydrate · 14 g sugar · 11 g fiber · 504 mg sodium · 292 mg calcium · 8 mg iron · 23 mg vitamin C · 6457 mcg beta-carotene · 2 mg vitamin E

Pizza Napolitano
Zi Caterina, Pompeii, Italy

MAKES 6 SERVINGS

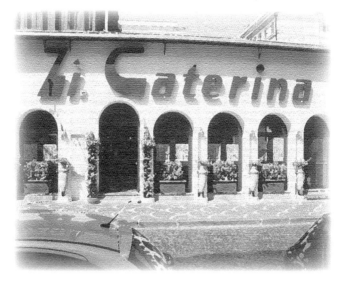

*I*n AD 79, the eruption of Mt. Vesuvius buried Pompeii under a deep blanket of volcanic ash. Today, archeologists are uncovering the well-preserved remains of the surprisingly modern town. A few steps away, scientists and tourists take a lunch break at Pompeii's best restaurant, Zi Caterina. Founded in 1920 by Giuseppe and Caterina Acanfora, and still run by the Acanfora family, the restaurant serves up authentic and delicious traditional meals.

Unlike American restaurants, which bury their pizzas under a lava of cheese, many Italian pizzas are completely cheeseless and, as a result, far healthier. At Zi Caterina, pizza chef Andrea Ruggiero uses oak logs in an oven that reaches 350°C. Home cooks can be a bit less ambitious.

3 medium tomatoes
2 tablespoons fresh oregano
2 tablespoons chopped fresh basil, divided
3 large garlic cloves

cornmeal for dusting pizza pan
1 15-inch premade or homemade pizza crust
pinch of sea salt (optional)

Preheat oven to 500°F.

Place 2 tomatoes, oregano, I tablespoon basil, and garlic into a food processor. Process until desired pizza sauce consistency. Dust a preheated pizza stone or pizza pan with a little bit of cornmeal to prevent sticking. Place pizza crust on top of the stone or pan. Spread pizza sauce evenly on the pizza crust. Chop remaining tomato and spread as a topping on the pizza. Bake for 12 to 15 minutes, until the edge of the crust starts to brown. Remove from oven and place remaining basil leaves on as a pizza topping. Bake for an additional 3 minutes, until the basil leaves begin to wilt. Remove from oven and sprinkle the top with a pinch of sea salt, if desired.

Per serving (1/6 of recipe): 199 calories · 4 g fat · 1 g saturated fat · 18% calories from fat · 0 mg cholesterol · 5 g protein · 35 g carbohydrate · 2 g sugar · 2 g fiber · 316 mg sodium · 24 mg calcium · 2 mg iron · 13 mg vitamin C · 194 mcg beta-carotene · 1 mg vitamin E

VEGETABLE GOULASH

Old Dungeon Ghyll Hotel, Cumbria, England

MAKES 15 TO 20 SERVINGS

1 tablespoon olive oil
2 red onions, chopped
10 cups vegetable broth
2 carrots, chopped
1 16-ounce can fava beans, drained and rinsed
3 celery stalks, finely chopped
1 large sweet potato, chopped
1 rutabaga, chopped
1 beet, chopped

1 16-ounce can kidney beans, drained and rinsed
1 cup chopped green beans
2 plum tomatoes, chopped
2 tablespoons caraway seeds
5 tablespoons Italian seasoning
salt, to taste
black pepper, to taste
2 tablespoons chopped fresh basil

Add the olive oil to a 16-quart pot and cook the onions for 5 to 8 minutes, stirring regularly. Add the other ingredients, except for the herbs and seasoning. Bring to a boil, then simmer on medium low for 15 to 20 minutes, until the vegetables are soft.

Turn off the heat and season with the caraway seeds, Italian seasoning, salt, and black pepper. Garnish with the fresh basil.

Per serving (1/15 of recipe): 109 calories · 1 g fat · 0.2 g saturated fat · 12% calories from fat · 0 mg cholesterol · 5 g protein · 21 g carbohydrate · 6 g sugar · 6 g fiber · 877 mg sodium · 78 mg calcium · 2 mg iron · 11 mg vitamin C · 1999 mcg beta-carotene · 1 mg vitamin E

Tofu Scallops with Truffled Bean Sprout Risotto

Coast, Vancouver, British Columbia

MAKES 6 SERVINGS

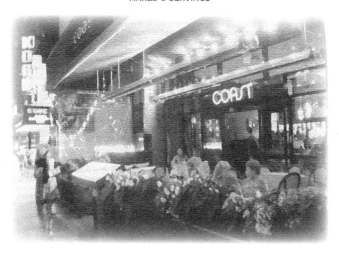

Coast's Chef de Cuisine, Pedro Gonzalez, knows how to whip up fancy and creative plant-based food at this seafood restaurant in Vancouver.

TRUFFLED BEAN SPROUT RISOTTO

4 teaspoons grape seed oil
4 teaspoons minced shallots
2 teaspoons minced garlic
1/2 cup white wine
4 cups finely chopped mung bean sprouts (minced to resemble Arborio rice)
1/2 cup vegetable broth
1/2 cup Cashew Cream (see recipe below)
1 teaspoon chopped black truffles
1/2 teaspoon Meyer lemon zest
kosher salt, to taste
white pepper, to taste
1 teaspoon chopped fresh parsley
1 teaspoon chopped fresh chives

SAUTÉED PEA TIPS

2 teaspoons grape seed oil
1 cup fresh pea tips (can substitute spinach)
kosher salt, to taste
white pepper, to taste

TOFU SCALLOPS

2 8-ounce blocks medium-firm tofu
kosher salt, to taste
white pepper, to taste
2 teaspoons grape seed oil

Truffled bean sprout risotto: In a sauté pan over medium heat, add the grape seed oil and shallots. Sweat the shallots until they begin to turn translucent. Add the garlic and sauté until lightly browned. Deglaze with white wine and reduce until almost dry. Next, add the bean sprouts and stir with a wooden spoon and continue to cook for 2 to 3 minutes. Add the broth and cashew cream (use more broth to thin out the cashew cream if necessary). Allow the cashew cream to set and cook out for about 5 to 8 minutes. Much like cornstarch, the cashew cream activates and serves as a thickening agent. Take the bean sprouts and cashew cream to a stage that resembles a creamy risotto and season with truffles, lemon zest, salt, white pepper, and finish with fresh parsley and chives.

Sautéed pea tips: In a sauté pan over medium heat, add the grape seed oil. Add the pea tips and sauté for 2 to 3 minutes until wilted and tender. Season with kosher salt and white pepper.

To assemble the plate of tofu scallops: With a round ring mold (3/4–inch to 1-inch diameter), cut out about 5 pieces from the blocks of tofu to resemble scallops. The size and shape of the tofu scallop can vary, depending on the individual's desired scallop size (small or large scallops/tall or short scallops). Season them generously with salt and white pepper. Sear the tofu in a hot sauté pan with grape seed oil.

Arrange the seared tofu scallops on the plate and spoon the risotto around the scallops. Top dish off with sautéed pea tips.

CASHEW CREAM
MAKES 2 1/4 CUPS

2 cups whole raw cashews   2 cups water

Soak the cashews overnight in water. Drain and place in a blender. Add water to cover the cashews. Blend until smooth. The consistency of the cashew cream should resemble that of heavy whipping cream. If more water is required, add more gradually and continue to blend.

Per serving (1/6 of recipe): 193 calories · 13 g fat · 2 g saturated fat · 60% calories from fat · 0 mg cholesterol · 9 g protein · 8 g carbohydrate · 3 g sugar · 2 g fiber · 542 mg sodium · 176 mg calcium · 3 mg iron · 9 mg vitamin C · 314 mcg beta-carotene · 2 mg vitamin E

WILD MUSHROOM AND PISTACHIO WELLINGTON
Alfresco, St. Ives, England

MAKES 4 SERVINGS

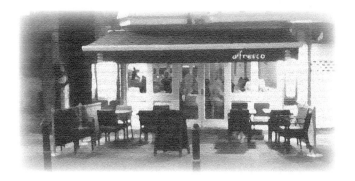

*S*t. Ives is a beautiful seaside town in western England, where Alfresco serves up delightfully healthful food.

1/4 cup finely chopped shallots
2 garlic cloves, crushed
2 1/2 tablespoons vegan margarine
8 ounces seasonal wild mushrooms, roughly chopped
1/2 cup cooking sherry
2 tablespoons chopped fresh tarragon

salt, to taste
black pepper, to taste
1/4 cup toasted pistachio nuts
8 ounces vegan puff pastry
1 tablespoon unsweetened non-dairy milk

Pan fry shallots and garlic with margarine over a low heat, until softened and golden. Add mushrooms and turn up heat until nicely browned. Add cooking sherry and tarragon. Cook until no liquid is visible in pan. Season with salt and black pepper to taste and leave to cool. Grind the pistachios in a food processor for a few seconds to break up. Add mushroom mixture and blitz, leaving a nice coarse texture.

Roll out pastry to 2 mm thickness, then cut into 4 equal squares. Divide mushroom mixture into 4 balls. Place on pastry, fold over and crimp edges. Brush with unsweetened non-dairy milk and bake for 20 minutes at 390°F. Serve with seasonal vegetables and tarragon jus.

Per serving (1/4 of recipe): 82 calories · 32 g fat · 7 g saturated fat · 58% calories from fat · 0 mg cholesterol · 8 g protein · 36 g carbohydrate · 3 g sugar · 3 g fiber · 555 mg sodium · 64 mg calcium · 4 mg iron · 5 mg vitamin C · 179 mcg beta-carotene · 2 mg vitamin E

PLUM'S SMOKEY MAC

Plum Bistro, Seattle, Washington

MAKES 14 SERVINGS

sea salt
1 pound elbow macaroni
8 ounces smoked tofu cut into thin strips
1 large yellow onion, chopped
4 garlic cloves, smashed and divided
leaves from 1/4 bunch fresh thyme
freshly ground black pepper
3 cups unsweetened soymilk
3 or 4 large thyme sprigs

3 tablespoons vegan margarine
3 tablespoons all-purpose flour
1 cup store-bought vegan mayonnaise
 or heavy soy cream
5 cups shredded mozzarella-style vegan
 cheese, divided
1/4 cup chopped flat-leaf parsley
1/2 cup panko bread crumbs
1–2 tablespoons crushed red pepper

Bring a pot of salted water to a boil over high heat. Add the macaroni and cook according to package directions until al dente, about 8 to 9 minutes. Drain.

Preheat the oven to 400°F.

Heat a sauté pan. Add the tofu and cook until crispy. Add onion, 2 garlic cloves, and thyme leaves and cook for about 5 minutes to soften the onion. Season with salt and black pepper. Remove from heat and set aside.

In a small saucepan heat the soymilk with the thyme sprigs and remaining 2 garlic cloves. Melt the margarine in a large, deep skillet over medium-high heat. Whisk in the flour and cook for about 1 minute, on medium-low (you do not want a dark sauce) stirring constantly, to keep lumps from forming. Strain the solids out of the soymilk and whisk it into the butter and flour mixture. Continue to whisk vigorously, and cook until the mixture is smooth. Stir in the tofu-onion mixture and vegan mayonnaise or heavy soy cream, continue to cook and stir to incorporate. Season with salt and black pepper. Add the cooked macaroni, 4 cups of the cheese, and the parsley, and fold to coat the macaroni with the cheese mixture. Scrape into a 3-quart baking dish and sprinkle with the remaining 1 cup cheese, panko bread crumbs, and crushed red pepper. Bake for 30 minutes, or until hot and bubbly.

Per serving (1/14 of recipe): 378 calories · 15 g fat · 3 g saturated fat · 34% calories from fat · 0 mg cholesterol · 17 g protein · 46 g carbohydrate · 12 g sugar · 3 g fiber · 821 mg sodium · 372 mg calcium · 3 mg iron · 4 mg vitamin C · 137 mcg beta-carotene · 1 mg vitamin E

ACORN SQUASH

National Press Club, Washington, District of Columbia

MAKES 2 SERVINGS

*O*n the fault line between politics and press, the National Press Club is where seismic events occur daily. Amid the acrimony of political clashes, where better to bury the hatchet than in The Fourth Estate's acorn squash?

ACORN SQUASH

1 acorn squash	1/8 teaspoon ground nutmeg
2 tablespoons maple syrup	dash of ground cloves
1/4 teaspoon ground cinnamon	

GRAIN MIX

1/2 cup dry brown rice	3 tablespoons dried cherries
1/4 cup dry wild rice	3 tablespoons pecans (halved)
3 tablespoons dried apricots	

2 cups apple cider	2 tablespoons vegetable broth
3 fresh thyme sprigs	salt, to taste
1 cup baby spinach	black pepper, to taste
1 cup Swiss chard	

Preheat oven to 350°F.

Cut acorn squash in half and scoop out seeds. Whisk together maple syrup, cinnamon, nutmeg, and cloves. Coat cut surface of acorn squash with maple syrup mixture. Roast for 45 minutes uncovered, cut side up in oven.

While squash is baking, cook brown and wild rice according to package directions.

For apple cider reduction, bring 2 cups of apple cider to a boil, then turn down to a simmer and add fresh thyme sprigs. Let simmer and thicken while squash and rice are cooking.

Julienne dried apricots and toast pecans for 2 minutes (watch carefully to not burn pecans). Set aside until rice is done.

A few minutes before squash and rice are done, chop and sauté spinach and Swiss chard in vegetable broth with a dash of salt and black pepper. Mix cooked brown and wild rice with julienned apricots, whole dried cherries, and toasted pecans. Remove squash

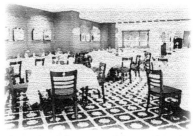

from oven and place each half cut side up in the center of 2 plates. Remove thyme from apple cider reduction and drizzle some over the cut squash halves. Stuff the squashes with the grain mixture and drizzle again with some of the apple cider reduction. Ring the sautéed greens around the edge of the squash and drizzle with remainder of the apple cider reduction. Serve.

Optional additions to add to the top of finished meal:
- Roast acorn squash seeds or use packaged pumpkin seeds and sprinkle over the top.
- *Cranberry garnish:* Use an immersion blender and blend 2 navel oranges and 1/4 cup frozen or fresh cranberries with a small amount of white sugar. Blend, but leave chunky.

Per serving (1/2 of recipe): 660 calories · 9 g fat · 1 g saturated fat · 12% calories from fat · 0 mg cholesterol · 12 g protein · 140 g carbohydrate · 57 g sugar · 17 g fiber · 273 mg sodium · 190 mg calcium · 5 mg iron · 26 mg vitamin C · 2123 mcg beta-carotene · 2 mg vitamin E

SPAGHETTI ARRABBIATA

Linus Bar Ristorante, Cannigione, Sardinia

MAKES 6 SERVINGS

1/4 cup olive oil
4 garlic cloves, minced
1/4 teaspoon cayenne pepper

1 15-ounce can diced tomatoes
8 ounces dry spaghetti

Heat olive oil in a pan over medium heat. Add garlic and cayenne pepper to oil and sauté, being careful the garlic does not brown, about 1 minute. Add diced tomatoes to pan. Turn down heat and allow the sauce to simmer for 10 to 12 minutes, stirring occasionally. Boil pasta according to package directions to al dente, drain, and rinse. Add pasta to the simmering tomato sauce, mix well, and simmer 3 to 5 minutes longer.

Per serving (1/6 of recipe): 263 calories · 10 g fat · 1 g saturated fat · 34% calories from fat · 0 mg cholesterol · 7 g protein · 36 g carbohydrate · 2 g sugar · 3 g fiber · 103 mg sodium · 33 mg calcium · 2 mg iron · 7 mg vitamin C · 66 mcg beta-carotene · 2 mg vitamin E

PEACH TOFU AND TEMPEH WITH CHARRED PURPLE BEANS

Plum Bistro, Seattle, Washington

MAKES 4 SERVINGS

2 overripe peaches
2 cups white wine
1 cup chopped fresh cilantro
2 tablespoons sugar
1/2 cup fresh lime juice (about 4 medium limes)
1 1/4 cups olive oil, divided
1 cup chipotle peppers in adobo sauce, minced

2/3 cup whole roasted garlic cloves, with a few pieces smashed
2 teaspoons salt, plus extra to taste for the beans
2 teaspoons black pepper, plus extra to taste for the beans
4 2-ounce slices tempeh
4 2-ounce slices tofu
2 teaspoons chopped fresh garlic
1 pound purple beans, trimmed

In a large bowl, smash the overripe peaches until the flesh comes off the pits in chunks. Add wine, cilantro, sugar, lime juice, 1 cup olive oil, chipotles, roasted garlic, salt, and black pepper. Mix well.

Pour a thin layer of the marinade on the bottom of a medium pan such as a 9 x 9-inch glass dish. Put the tempeh and tofu on top, and then pour the remaining marinade over it. Cover and store in the refrigerator 5 to 6 hours, or overnight for a stronger flavor.

In a large frying pan, heat the remaining 1/4 cup olive oil over high heat. Add the fresh garlic and cook briefly, stirring with a wooden spoon or spatula until the garlic begins to brown. Add the beans. Shake to turn them, or turn them with tongs, and cook for a moment until the other side begins to char at the edges. Remove from heat and season the beans with salt and black pepper to taste.

Heat a medium sauté pan or flat-top griddle over medium heat. Cook the marinated tofu and tempeh slices until golden brown. Spoon the marinade onto tofu and tempeh as it is cooking in the sauté pan for a more intense flavor. Arrange the slices on top of the beans.

Per serving (1/4 of recipe): 1001 calories · 77 g fat · 11 g saturated fat · 67% calories from fat · 0 mg cholesterol · 19 g protein · 48 g carbohydrate · 23 g sugar · 8 g fiber · 2153 mg sodium · 251 mg calcium · 5 mg iron · 39 mg vitamin C · 1133 mcg beta-carotene · 12 mg vitamin E

LINGUINE WITH TRUFFLE PESTO AND PORCINI MUSHROOMS

Ristorante Al Porta, Sardinia

MAKES 4 SERVINGS

8 ounces dry linguine
1 3/4 cups dried porcini mushrooms
2 cups water
2 tablespoons olive oil
1 large garlic clove, minced
1/4 teaspoon salt, plus more to taste

1/4 teaspoon black pepper
1/4 cup coconut milk coffee creamer
2 drops truffle oil
chopped green onions, for garnish (optional)

Bring large stockpot of salted water to boil. Add linguine and cook according to package directions until al dente, about 8 minutes. Drain; do not rinse.

Reconstitute mushrooms by bringing 2 cups water to boil. Add mushrooms and boil for 2 to 4 minutes, until mushrooms are softened. Drain, then pat dry. Chop mushrooms into medium pieces, about 1/2 inch.

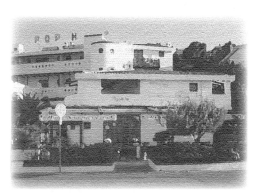

Slowly heat olive oil in large sauté pan. Add garlic and cook over medium-low heat for 45 seconds. Add salt, black pepper, and chopped mushrooms, raise temperature to medium and cook for 4 minutes. Slowly stir in coconut creamer and lower temperature. Cook, stirring occasionally, for 3 minutes. Add truffle oil, then linguine. Stir to coat pasta, then season to taste with salt and black pepper.

Top with chopped green onions for garnish, if desired.

Per serving (1/4 of recipe): 361 calories · 8 g fat · 1 g saturated fat · 20% calories from fat · 0 mg cholesterol · 11 g protein · 62 g carbohydrate · 4 g sugar · 4 g fiber · 524 mg sodium · 16 mg calcium · 2 mg iron · 1 mg vitamin C · 1 mcg beta-carotene · 1 mg vitamin E

CASADO

Soda 13 Por 2, Hojancha, Costa Rica

MAKES 4 SERVINGS

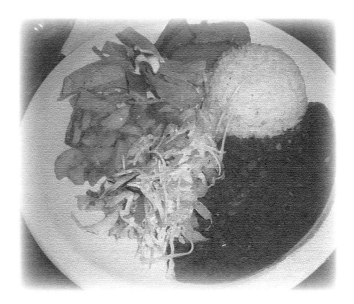

*T*he sign says only "Soda 13 Por 2" and, aside from the proprietor's friendly welcome, the restaurant is unremarkable at first glance. But the village of Hojancha is the epicenter of a "blue zone"—one of the handful of places on Earth where people live extraordinarily long lives. The others, described in Dan Buettner's book, *Blue Zones*, are Okinawa, Japan; Loma Linda, California; Sardinia, Italy; and Ikaria, Greece.

Much of the credit goes to the local cuisine, typified by the Casado, a generous plate of black beans, rice, a vegetable, and sweet plantano (plantains), to which meat may or may not be added.

By the way, in Costa Rica, a "soda" is a small café and Casado comes from the word for a man who, being happily married, stays in his casa, presumably eating simple, healthful food.

2 cups water	1 whole onion
1 cup dry rice	2 garlic cloves
1 15-ounce can black beans	1 celery stalk

FOR CABBAGE SALAD

2 cups very finely shredded white cabbage

1 tomato, seeded and chopped

3 tablespoons chopped fresh cilantro

1/4 red bell pepper, chopped

1/4 cup lime juice

4 teaspoons agave or maple syrup

kosher salt, to taste

1 small carrot, grated using the larger holes on a box grater

minced hot peppers or Italian peppers, to taste (optional)

1 tablespoon canola oil

2 ripe plantains (nearly black with some remaining yellow spots)

4 flour tortillas

To make rice and beans: Bring water to boil. Add rice. Bring back to boil, cover, and simmer on low for 20 minutes.

Empty can of beans, with liquid, into a small pot. Peel the onion (keeping it whole) and garlic and cut celery into 4 pieces. Place vegetables in pot with beans and bring to a boil. Cover pot and turn to medium low. Cook for 15 minutes. Drain when done. Remove the onion, garlic, and celery.

To make cabbage salad: In a bowl, combine cabbage, tomato, cilantro, and bell pepper. Toss to combine. In a small bowl, mix together lime juice, agave, and salt just before serving, and toss to combine. Add shredded carrots, and minced hot peppers or Italian peppers, if using.

To make plantains: Heat canola oil in a medium skillet over medium heat. Peel plantains, cut lengthwise, then crosswise. This will give you 4 pieces per plantain. Place cut side down in skillet and cook until brown, about 3 minutes. Flip and cook on the other side for 3 minutes. Remove from pan.

Keeping pan on the burner, place a tortilla in the skillet. Let sit for 30 seconds or so, just until browned on one side. Flip and cook on other side until browned. Repeat with remaining tortillas.

On each plate, place roughly one cup of rice with beans next to it.

Fill plate with 2 pieces of plantain, a folded tortilla, and a serving of cabbage salad.

Per serving (1/4 of recipe): 647 calories · 8 g fat · 1 g saturated fat · 11% calories from fat · 0 mg cholesterol · 16 g protein · 133 g carbohydrate · 28 g sugar · 14 g fiber · 789 mg sodium · 143 mg calcium · 6 mg iron · 42 mg vitamin C · 1783 mcg beta-carotene · 1 mg vitamin E

Ravioli with Porcini Mushrooms and Artichokes

Ristorante Al Porto, Sardinia

MAKES 2 SERVINGS

On Sardinia's rugged eastern coast, Cala Gonone is a haven for rock climbers, divers, and hikers. After a day's adventures, Al Porto offers a glass of wine and a hearty meal.

1 fresh artichoke
water
salt
8 ounces vegan butternut squash ravioli
2 tablespoons olive oil

2 garlic cloves, chopped
1 ounce dried porcini mushrooms, soaked in 1 cup water for 20 minutes, then drained

Trim 1 inch off top of fresh artichoke. Trim bottom stem, leaving 1 to 2 inches. With a pair of scissors, snip away pointy tips of artichoke leaves. Wash under running water to make sure all leaf tips are flushed out.

Pour 3 inches of water in medium pot, place steamer in pot, and bring water to boil. When water boils, place artichoke in steamer, cover, and steam for 25 to 40 minutes. Check water levels as you cook; if more is needed, pour in one cup and cover pot again. Artichoke is done with leaves pull off easily and meat at bottom of leaf is tender.

When artichoke is done, remove from steamer and plunge into bowl filled with ice water to stop the cooking process. After 2 minutes, remove artichoke from ice water and drain well. Peel away leaves until you reach artichoke heart. Trim stray hairs away from heart. Cut heart into 6 to 8 pieces. Scrape out any remaining pieces of heart and place with chopped pieces, again checking for hairs or fibrous pieces.

Bring 2 quarts of salted water to boil in large pot. When water boils, add ravioli and cook over low boil until ravioli floats to top, between 5 to 7 minutes. Remove from heat, reserving 3 tablespoons cooking water. Drain ravioli.

In medium saucepan, heat olive oil over medium heat, and then add garlic, artichoke pieces, and porcini mushrooms. Sauté for 3 to 4 minutes. Add 3 tablespoons cooking water, then place ravioli in pan and cook for 1 minute or less, making sure that ravioli doesn't stick to pan.

Remove from pan, spoon mushroom mixture over ravioli, and serve immediately.

Per serving (1/2 of recipe): 399 calories · 15 g fat · 2 g saturated fat · 33% calories from fat · 0 mg cholesterol · 10 g protein · 58 g carbohydrate · 1 g sugar · 6 g fiber · 160 mg sodium · 24 mg calcium · 2 mg iron · 4 mg vitamin C · 512 mcg beta-carotene · 2 mg vitamin E

RAVIOLI WITH TRUFFLES AND CELERIAC
Pan Dei, Saint-Tropez, France

MAKES 5 SERVINGS

This delightful recipe includes ingredients that are more familiar in France than elsewhere, but are good to get to know. Celeriac is a relative of common celery, but it is the root—not the stems and leaves—that are commonly eaten. Truffle juice (distinct from truffle oil) adds an earthy flavor to dishes and is commercially available at specialty shops and online.

9 ounces truffle juice
salt, to taste
14 tablespoons vegan margarine
1 celeriac root, chopped

3 1/2 ounces black truffles, chopped
1 packet ravioli dough (10 cm x 10 cm)
1 tablespoon olive oil

Heat 3 1/2 ounces of truffle juice, salt, and 10 tablespoons of margarine. When melted, add the celeriac. Stir frequently over a low flame until the celeriac is cooked, about 15 minutes. Add the truffles and cook for an additional 10 minutes. Adjust the seasoning to taste. Remove the chopped vegetables from the pan.

Spread out the ravioli squares and, using a brush, lightly spread olive oil on both sides. Add 1 teaspoon of the chopped vegetable mixture and close the ravioli, taking care to eliminate trapped air. Store in freezer if not using immediately.

To prepare the sauce, bring 5 1/2 ounces of truffle juice to a boil, then remove from heat, add 4 tablespoons margarine, and mix until the sauce thickens.

Thaw the ravioli if frozen, then immerse in boiling water. The ravioli will float to the top of the pot when it's finished. Drain and finish cooking in the sauce for 2 minutes.

Place on plates, decorate with truffle slices if desired, and enjoy!

Per serving (1/5 of recipe): 552 calories · 31 g fat · 6 g saturated fat · 50% calories from fat · 0 mg cholesterol · 11 g protein · 58 g carbohydrate · 3 g sugar · 5 g fiber · 1326 mg sodium · 67 mg calcium · 5 mg iron · 8 mg vitamin C · 202 mcg beta-carotene · 3 mg vitamin E

Vegetables and Grains

BESAN KE GATTE
Imperial Palace, Rajkot, Gujarat, India

MAKES 4 SERVINGS

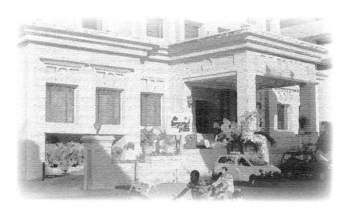

*T*he Imperial Palace is a luxury hotel in Rajkot, Gujarat.

DOUGH

1 cup besan (gram or chickpea flour)
1/2 teaspoon baking powder
1/2 teaspoon salt
1 tablespoon dried coriander
1/2 teaspoon red chili powder
1/2 teaspoon turmeric powder
1 1/2 tablespoons crushed coriander

seeds
1 1/2 tablespoons ginger-garlic paste
   (or finely minced ginger and garlic)
1/2 cup olive oil
4 1/2 tablespoons plain soy yogurt
1 tablespoon oil for frying

GRAVY

7 tablespoons vegan margarine
2 teaspoons whole garam masala
   (cloves, cinnamon, bay leaf,
   cardamom)
1 teaspoon cumin seeds
1/2 teaspoon asafetida
7 tablespoons chopped onion
1 1/2 tablespoons ginger-garlic paste

1/2 cup chopped tomato
1 teaspoon red chili powder
1 teaspoon turmeric
1 teaspoon coriander powder
1 cup plain soy yogurt
salt, to taste
3/4 cup water
fresh cilantro, for garnish (optional)

For the dough: In a medium bowl, mix all of the dry ingredients together. Add the ginger-garlic paste. Make a tight dough using olive oil and soy yogurt. Boil water in a large pan. Make 6-inch long rolls of dough. Place in boiling water and cook until firm. Drain water, then remove cooked dough and cut into small pieces. In a small pan, heat oil over medium-low heat and fry dough rounds ("gatte") in 1 tablespoon oil until lightly browned.

For the gravy: Heat margarine in medium pan over medium-high heat. Add whole garam masala, cumin seeds, and asafetida. Add onion, frying until golden brown, then ginger-garlic paste. Add tomato and stir-fry until cooked. Add red chili powder, turmeric, coriander, then soy yogurt. Stir and cook for 5 minutes. Add salt to taste. Add 3/4 cup water and bring to a boil.

Once water has incorporated into the sauce, add the fried gatte. Garnish with fresh coriander, if desired.

Per serving (1/4 of recipe): 559 calories · 51 g fat · 8 g saturated fat · 75% calories from fat · 0 mg cholesterol · 9 g protein · 29 g carbohydrate · 9 g sugar · 5 g fiber · 730 mg sodium · 205 mg calcium · 4 mg iron · 21 mg vitamin C · 359 mcg beta-carotene · 6 mg vitamin E

WHOLE-WHEAT BREAD
Old Dungeon Ghyll Hotel, Cumbria, England

MAKES 3 LOAVES (14 SLICES PER LOAF)

14 cups whole-wheat flour	(use more if you like sweeter bread)
1 tablespoon salt	1/2 cup olive oil
7 cups water	3 packets yeast (3/4 ounce total), not
1/4 cup sugar, brown sugar, or molasses	dissolved in water

Mix flour and salt in a large bowl. In a separate bowl, mix the water, sugar, oil, and yeast with a whisk. Pour into flour. Knead until very springy (push fingers into the dough to test). Cover the bowl with plastic wrap and let rise for two hours. Place the dough into 3 loaf pans. Bake at 150°F for 20 minutes, then at 325°F for 30 minutes.

Per serving (2 slices): 330 calories · 7 g fat · 1 g saturated fat · 19% calories from fat · 0 mg cholesterol · 11 g protein · 60 g carbohydrate · 3 g sugar · 9 g fiber · 342 mg sodium · 30 mg calcium · 3 mg iron · 0 mg vitamin C · 4 mcg beta-carotene · 1 mg vitamin E

CHARRED BROCCOLINI

Plum Bistro, Seattle, Washington

MAKES 4 SERVINGS

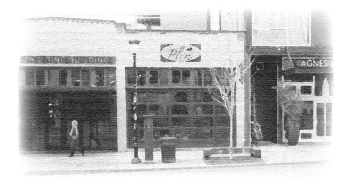

3/4 pound broccolini
1/4 cup olive oil
1/2 medium red bell pepper, cut into julienne strips
1 tablespoon chopped fresh garlic

1 medium lemon, halved and seeds removed
1/2 teaspoon crushed red pepper, or more to taste
sea salt, to taste
black pepper, to taste

Trim stalk ends of broccolini. Wash, and then dry thoroughly.

Heat olive oil over high heat, and then add bell pepper. Cook for 1 minute, stirring with a wooden spoon until pepper starts to sizzle. Add garlic and cook for 25 to 30 seconds. Add broccolini and toss with tongs so that everything is covered with oil. Cook on one side for 1 minute or until bottom starts to char. Flip with tongs and cook other side for 1 to 2 minutes, shaking pan or flipping with tongs to evenly cook the broccolini.

After a minute or 2, when broccolini starts to wilt, squeeze lemon juice over the vegetables. Just a few gentle squeezes of the lemon will do. The pan will start to smoke, adding to the flavor. Sprinkle with crushed red pepper and season with sea salt and black pepper to taste. Toss one more time, remove from pan, and serve.

Per serving (1/4 of recipe): 158 calories · 14 g fat · 2 g saturated fat · 78% calories from fat · 0 mg cholesterol · 2 g protein · 8 g carbohydrate · 2 g sugar · 3 g fiber · 182 mg sodium · 40 mg calcium · 1 mg iron · 81 mg vitamin C · 1019 mcg beta-carotene · 4 mg vitamin E

PASTEL DE MAÍZ

Krystal Restaurant, Tenerife, Spain

MAKES 6 TO 8 SERVINGS

2 large ears of corn
3/4 cup chopped leeks
1/2 cup chopped onion
1/2 cup plus 1 tablespoon canola oil, divided
1/4 cup shredded vegan mozzarella cheese

1/2 cup vegan sour cream
few pinches salt
black pepper, to taste
1/2 tablespoon unsweetened non-dairy milk
1/3 cup corn meal

Preheat oven to 350°F. Remove husks from corn. Steam for 20 minutes or until tender. Rinse the corn with water until it cool enough to handle.

Cut the kernels off. Pulse the corn in food processor until roughly chopped.

Sauté the leeks and onion in 1 tablespoon canola oil over medium heat for 5 minutes.

Mix the corn, cheese, and sour cream with the onion-leek mixture. Add salt and black pepper and set aside.

Combine non-dairy milk and remaining 1/2 cup canola oil in a mixing bowl. Add corn meal. Mix thoroughly. Add corn mixture to mixing bowl. Mix thoroughly.

Spread entire mixture into a lightlyoiled 8 x 2-inch baking dish. Place baking dish inside a larger baking dish filled with hot water. Bake for 45 minutes, or until a knife placed in the center comes out mostly clean.

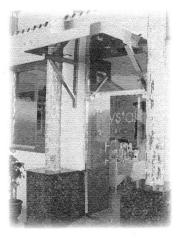

Per serving (1/6 of recipe): 309 calories · 26 g fat · 5 g saturated fat · 73% calories from fat · 0 mg cholesterol · 4 g protein · 18 g carbohydrate · 4 g sugar · 2 g fiber · 211 mg sodium · 10 mg calcium · 1 mg iron · 3 mg vitamin C · 66 mcg beta-carotene · 4 mg vitamin E

SWEET POTATO PURÉE

Pan Dei, Saint-Tropez, France

MAKES 6 SERVINGS

1 pound sweet potatoes, unpeeled
1 pound small white potatoes, unpeeled
salt, to taste

1 cup non-dairy milk of choice
8 tablespoons vegan margarine

Wash the sweet potatoes and potatoes, place in a pot, and cover with water. Add salt. Bring to boil and simmer for 30 minutes or until done. Drain. Peel the sweet potatoes and potatoes. Purée with a fork or a traditional food mill. Meanwhile, bring the non-dairy milk to a boil in a separate pan. Return the potatoes to the pot and stir over low heat with a wooden spoon for 2 to 3 minutes. Add margarine (in pieces), then the hot milk, bit by bit, stirring constantly. Finish by stirring with a whisk to a smooth consistency.

Per serving (1/6 of recipe): 232 calories · 13 g fat · 3 g saturated fat · 51% calories from fat · 0 mg cholesterol · 3 g protein · 26 g carbohydrate · 6 g sugar · 3 g fiber · 441 mg sodium · 86 mg calcium · 2 mg iron · 17 mg vitamin C · 5671 mcg beta-carotene · 2 mg vitamin E

HOW TO SELECT THE FRESHEST VEGETABLES

*G*iuliano Tortoriello gives his tips on selecting the very best and freshest vegetables. He owns Faraglioni, but he chooses the vegetables himself.

Asparagus: Bypass the white asparagus that people choose mainly for its appearance. For the best taste, choose green asparagus, especially the relatively small stalks. They should be soft to the touch, without any brownish parts.

Spinach: For a fresh taste, it should be purchased within 4 to 5 hours of harvest, and should be bright green and dry to the touch. Spinach deteriorates as time goes by.

Carrots: Favor small carrots. Big ones are too woody.

Green beans: Again, there is an advantage to smaller sizes. If they are too large, they will be stringy. Go for a bright green color.

Desserts

ALMOND PEACH TART

Elizabeth's Gone Raw, Washington, District of Columbia

MAKES 12 SERVINGS

1 pint almond, vanilla, peach, or strawberry non-dairy ice cream

6 peaches

SYRUP

1 teaspoon saffron threads
1 tablespoon water
1/2 cup light agave syrup

2 teaspoons finely cut fresh thyme
pinch of sea salt

ALMOND COOKIE

1 1/2 cups coconut flour
3/4 cup almond flour
2 tablespoons maple sugar or dark
  brown sugar
1 tablespoon ground flaxseeds
1/4 cup coconut butter

1/3 cup maple syrup
1/3 cup almond milk or other non-
  dairy milk
1/2 cup banana puree (1 or 2 bananas)
1 tablespoon almond extract
1 tablespoon vanilla extract

This recipe uses an oven at 200°F or a dehydrator at 115°F. If using oven, preheat to 200°F.

For the syrup: Soak the saffron threads in 1 tablespoon of water for 1 to 12 hours.

Combine agave, thyme, saffron threads and soaking water, and sea salt in a very large bowl. Mix well.

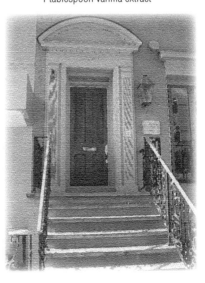

Slice peaches into wedges. If using dehydrator, peel peaches and slice into halves. Add the sliced peaches to the syrup and gently fold to coat the peach slices with syrup. Save any leftover agave syrup mixture.

Place peach slices on a lightly greased cookie sheet (or sheet covered with aluminum foil). Place the cookie sheet on a bottom-middle oven rack. Bake at 200°F for 4 hours, flipping slices after 2 hours. If using dehydrator, dehydrate at 115°F for 4 hours.

For the almond cookie: Combine coconut flour, almond flour, maple sugar, and ground flaxseeds in a medium bowl. Whisk, sift, or stir to combine well.

Add coconut butter, maple syrup, non-dairy milk, banana puree, almond extract, and vanilla extract to flour mixture. Combine well with a spatula and with hand kneading. The dough will be thick and crumbly.

Spread the dough on a lightly greased cookie sheet (or sheet covered with parchment paper). Using your hands or a rolling pin, spread the dough to about 1/4-inch thickness. If using de-hydrator, spread dough on dehydrator screen to about 1/4-inch thickness.

Place almond cookie sheet on an oven rack towards the top of the oven. For best results, use an insulated cookie sheet or ensure there is an additional cookie sheet below the almond cookie (the sheet with the peaches). Bake 3 1/2 hours at 200°F. If using dehydrator, dehydrate at 115°F for 4 to 6 hours.

Carefully slice the almond cookie into 2 x 4-inch rectangles. The cookies will be crumbly.

Layer several slices of baked peach, or one dehydrated peach half, onto each almond cookie. Use leftover agave syrup mixture to dress the plate or top the dessert. Serve with non-dairy ice cream.

Per serving (1/12 of recipe): 306 calories · 12 g fat · 5 g saturated fat · 32% calories from fat · 0 mg cholesterol · 5 g protein · 46 g carbohydrate · 35 g sugar · 8 g fiber · 133 mg sodium · 50 mg calcium · 3 mg iron · 8 mg vitamin C · 128 mcg beta-carotene · 3 mg vitamin E

PASSION FRUIT CAKE

Hotel Capitan Suizo, Tamarindo, Costa Rica

MAKES 12 SERVINGS

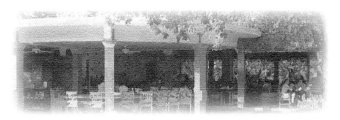

CAKE

1 1/2 cups flour
1 cup sugar
1 teaspoon baking soda
1/2 teaspoon salt

1/2 cup canola oil
1 cup non-dairy milk
1 tablespoon vanilla extract
1 tablespoon white distilled vinegar

PASSION FRUIT MOUSSE

3/4 cup sugar
14 ounces frozen passion fruit pulp

1 tablespoon agar flakes
1 12-ounce aseptic box silken firm tofu

For the cake: Preheat oven to 350°F. Grease a 9-inch cake pan. Whisk together flour, sugar, baking soda, and salt. Add oil, non-dairy milk, and vanilla. Mix until there are no lumps. Add vinegar and stir just until incorporated. Bake for 30 minutes or until a fork comes out clean.

For the mousse: Pour sugar and fruit pulp into a saucepan. Sprinkle in agar flakes, mix, and let sit for 10 minutes. Open box of tofu and put in the food processor or blender.

Slowly bring the fruit-agar mixture to a boil, stirring occasionally. Boil gently for 1 minute, remove from the heat, and let sit for a minute.

Pour liquid into food processor or blender and blend until smooth. Chill for an hour.

Spread the mousse on the cake. Cover and place in the refrigerator for 3 to 4 hours.

Per serving (1/12 of recipe): 312 calories · 11 g fat · 1 g saturated fat · 30% calories from fat · 0 mg cholesterol · 5 g protein · 51 g carbohydrate · 34 g sugar · 4 g fiber · 233 mg sodium · 41 mg calcium · 2 mg iron · 10 mg vitamin C · 261 mcg beta-carotene · 2 mg vitamin E

BLACKOUT PIE

Plant, Asheville, North Carolina

MAKES ONE 9-INCH PIE

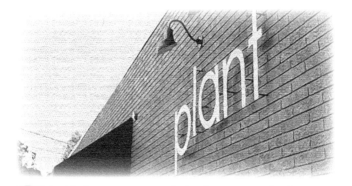

$\mathcal{T}$he blackout pie is one of Plant's most popular desserts.

CRUST

1/2 cup finely ground almonds
1 3/4 cups all-purpose flour
3/4 cup cocoa powder

3/4 cup sugar
5 ounces vegan margarine, melted

FILLING

1 16-ounce block silken tofu
3/4 cup brown sugar
3/4 cup powdered sugar
1 cup peanut butter

2 teaspoons vanilla extract
1 1/2 teaspoons salt
3/4 cup cocoa powder
10 tablespoons chocolate chips, melted

For the crust: Combine the almonds, flour, cocoa powder, and sugar in a large bowl and mix. Add the melted margarine, remix to make uniform, and cool. Press evenly into a greased 9-inch spring form pan and chill.

For the filling: Combine the tofu, sugars, peanut butter, vanilla, salt, and cocoa powder in a food processor and blend until very smooth. Add the melted chocolate and re-blend until smooth and uniform.

Using an offset spatula, add the filling to the chilled crust, and spread evenly. Chill the pie for at least 2 hours before serving.

Per serving (1/8 of pie): 734 calories · 39 g fat · 10 g saturated fat · 45% calories from fat · 0 mg cholesterol · 20 g protein · 91 g carbohydrate · 54 g sugar · 10 g fiber · 744 mg sodium · 92 mg calcium · 5 mg iron · 0 mg vitamin C · 90 mcg beta-carotene · 5 mg vitamin E

Fresh Fruit with Crème Anglais

Escopazzo, Miami, Florida

MAKES 15 SERVINGS

1 1/2 cups raw cashews
2 tablespoons agave nectar
juice of 1 lemon
1 vanilla bean, split lengthwise, or 2
   teaspoons pure vanilla extract

cinnamon (optional)
nutmeg (optional)
more sweetener (optional)

Soak the cashews in water for approximately 5 hours. Rinse nuts, drain, and process in a blender until creamy and smooth. Add the agave, lemon juice, vanilla, and cinnamon and nutmeg, if using. Mix until smooth. Taste, and if needed, add more sweetener. Add water until a rich, creamy consistency is reached.

Chill until ready to serve with any seasonal fresh fruit and chopped mint.

Per serving (1/15 of recipe, crème only): 81 calories · 6 g fat · 1 g saturated fat · 58% calories from fat · 0 mg cholesterol · 2 g protein · 6 g carbohydrate · 3 g sugar · 0.4 g fiber · 2 mg sodium · 5 mg calcium · 1 mg iron · 1 mg vitamin C · 0 mcg beta-carotene · 0.1 mg vitamin E

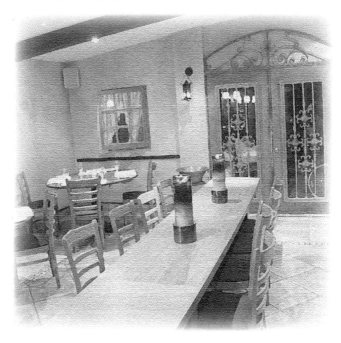

OATMEAL SHAKE

Irazu, Chicago, Illinois

MAKES 1 SERVING

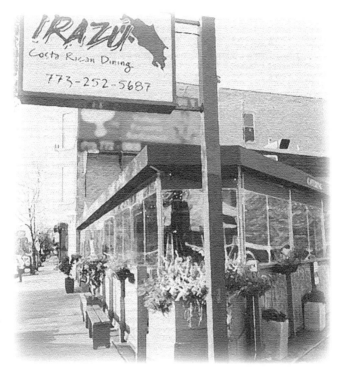

$\mathcal{T}$his recipe from Chef Cerdas-Salazar of Irazu in Chicago is simple and delicious.

1 cup almond milk*
1/4 cup rolled oats
dash of cinnamon
1/2 teaspoon vanilla extract

1/2–1 teaspoon agave nectar or other
    sweetener
5 ice cubes

Place all ingredients in blender and blend on high until very smooth.

If you are using sweetened almond milk, you may want to eliminate the agave.

Per serving: 132 calories · 4 g fat · 0.5 g saturated fat · 28% calories from fat · 0 mg cholesterol · 4 g protein · 19 g carbohydrate · 3 g sugar · 3 g fiber · 186 mg sodium · 216 mg calcium · 1 mg iron · 0 mg vitamin C · 0 mcg beta-carotene · 10 mg vitamin E

RAW KEY LIME TART

Six Main, Chester, Connecticut

MAKES 8 SERVINGS

CRUST

3/4 cup pumpkin seeds or walnuts

15 Medjool dates, pitted and roughly chopped

3/4 teaspoon cinnamon

3/4 teaspoon salt

FILLING

1 cup key lime juice or 1 cup freshly squeezed lime juice

3 avocados, halved, pitted, and skin removed

1 1/2 cups agave nectar or maple syrup

1 1/4 cups coconut oil (warm in microwave in 10 second intervals until it melts)

2 tablespoons soy lecithin granules

fresh lime slice, for garnish (optional)

1/8 teaspoon sugar, for garnish (optional)

To make the crust: Process seeds or nuts in food processor until finely chopped. Add dates, cinnamon, and salt, and process until well incorporated and crust sticks together when pressed between your fingers.

Press down into an 11-inch tart or spring form pan, making sure that the crust is spread evenly throughout bottom and sides.

Chill in refrigerator while making key lime filling.

For filling: Place all filling ingredients in food processor and blend until smooth, about 3 minutes. After 3 minutes, scrape sides and bottom of food processor to catch any stray pieces of avocado. Process 2 minutes longer.

Pour 1/4 to 1/2 cup into tart crust; if there are any chunky parts, spread lightly on bottom of crust and process remaining filling for 1 minute longer. Pour remaining filling into chilled crust, cover tightly with plastic wrap, and chill in refrigerator for 3 to 4 hours or overnight. Release from pan and serve.

Optional garnish: Take a thin slice of lime, cut halfway through and twist, pressing it slightly into middle of tart. Sprinkle lightly with 1/8 teaspoon sugar.

Per serving (1/8 of recipe): 676 calories · 48 g fat · 32 g saturated fat · 61% calories from fat · 0 mg cholesterol · 5 g protein · 66 g carbohydrate · 56 g sugar · 6 g fiber · 233 mg sodium · 24 mg calcium · 1 mg iron · 7 mg vitamin C · 37 mcg beta-carotene · 1 mg vitamin E

CHOCOLATE SOY FLAN

Fairmont Vancouver Airport, Vancouver, British Columbia

MAKES 6 SERVINGS

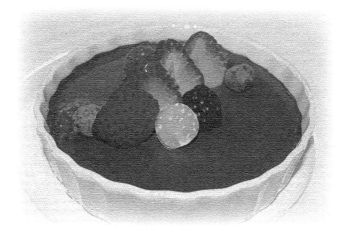

*G*uests choose it because it is literally steps from their departure gates. But they are surprised that this luxury hotel features a full vegan menu, including this delightful chocolate soy flan.

16 fluid ounces chocolate soymilk
1/2 cup fresh berries

1 pound dairy-free dark chocolate (in small pieces)

Heat the soymilk in a medium pot to just under a boil and pour over the chocolate pieces. Whisk together until the chocolate is completely melted. Pour warm ganache mixture into ramekin or serving vessel of your choice. Garnish with fresh berries.

Per serving (1/6 of recipe): 468 calories · 25 g fat · 14 g saturated fat · 48% calories from fat · 0 mg cholesterol · 6 g protein · 55 g carbohydrate · 43 g sugar · 6 g fiber · 61 mg sodium · 146 mg calcium · 7 mg iron · 8 mg vitamin C · 22 mcg beta-carotene · 0.5 mg vitamin E

Panna Cotta with Strawberry Ragout

Kopps, Berlin, Germany

MAKES 4 SERVINGS

13 1/2 fluid ounces soy creamer
3 tablespoons agave nectar
1 teaspoon agar powder

1 vanilla bean
1 1/2 cups strawberries
1 1/2 tablespoons raw cane sugar

In a saucepan, mix the soy creamer with the agave nectar and agar powder. Cut the vanilla bean lengthwise and scratch out the vanilla seeds with a knife. Add the seeds as well as the pod to the cream mixture and slowly heat, constantly stirring, until it starts to boil. The cream needs to boil for at least a minute so that the agar can thicken the mixture properly. Remove from heat.

Prepare 4 ramekins by rinsing them with cold water.

Remove the vanilla bean pod from the panna cotta and fill the prepared ramekins with the mixture. Cover and cool for at least 4 hours in the refrigerator.

Meanwhile, rinse the strawberries, remove the stems, and cut each berry into four pieces. Marinate with sugar in a small bowl.

Turn each ramekin upside down over a plate for a pretty presentation of the panna cotta. Arrange strawberry ragout around panna cotta and serve.

Per serving (1/4 of recipe): 190 calories · 7 g fat · 0.5 g saturated fat · 33% calories from fat · 0 mg cholesterol · 2 g protein · 31 g carbohydrate · 28 g sugar · 1 g fiber · 28 mg sodium · 23 mg calcium · 0.6 mg iron · 32 mg vitamin C · 20 mcg beta-carotene · 1 mg vitamin E

Breakfasts

BREAKFAST SCRAMBLE

Blossom, New York, New York

MAKES 4 SERVINGS

*A*s elegant as its name, Blossom is a garden of delicious flavors.

SUN-DRIED TOMATO RELISH

10 tablespoons sun-dried tomatoes
1/4 cup fresh basil
3 large tomatoes, cut into quarters
2 tablespoons olive oil

1/2 teaspoon salt
1/8 teaspoon black pepper
juice of 1/2 lemon

2 pounds firm or extra-firm tofu
1 teaspoon turmeric
5 tablespoons nutritional yeast
1 teaspoon salt

1/4 teaspoon black pepper
2 teaspoons tamari
1 tablespoon vegan margarine

Place all relish ingredients together in a food processor or blender and mix for a few seconds.

Combine relish with tofu, turmeric, nutritional yeast, salt, black pepper, and tamari. Make sure to combine with your hands, not a fork or spoon, until mixture is broken into small bits.

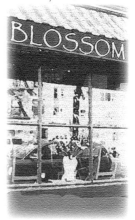

Sauté mixture in a pan with vegan margarine over medium heat. Serve in a whole-grain tortilla as a wrap, or on a plate with whole-grain toast.

Per serving (1/4 of recipe): 333 calories · 20 g fat · 4 g saturated fat · 51% calories from fat · 0 mg cholesterol · 27 g protein · 20 g carbohydrate · 8 g sugar · 8 g fiber · 1292 mg sodium · 494 mg calcium · 6 mg iron · 24 mg vitamin C · 723 mcg beta-carotene · 2 mg vitamin E

Breakfast Tamale

Radical Eats, Houston, Texas

MAKES 12 TAMALES

*H*ouston is home to this Mexican-inspired breakfast tamale. It will start your day off right.

MASA

2 cups vegetable broth	1 teaspoon sea salt
2 cups masa (corn flour)	3/4 teaspoon baking powder
1 14-ounce can whole peeled tomatoes	1/2 cup olive oil
1 teaspoon chopped fresh sage	

FILLING

2 cups crumbled firm tofu	2 tablespoons nutritional yeast
2 tablespoons chopped onion	2 tablespoons lemon juice
2 tablespoons chopped red bell pepper	1/2 teaspoon minced garlic
1 tablespoon red miso	1 teaspoon sea salt
1 tablespoon yellow mustard	1 teaspoon black pepper

12 soaked corn husks or 8 x 8-inch squares of tin foil for rolling.

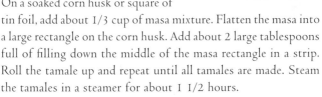

For the masa: Heat the vegetable broth in a pot over high heat. Add piping hot vegetable broth to masa in a food processor. Mix until all is integrated. Add the tomatoes, sage, salt, and baking powder. Integrate completely, then add the oil. Mix for 3 minutes.

For the filling: Mix all of the filling ingredients in a large bowl.

On a soaked corn husk or square of tin foil, add about 1/3 cup of masa mixture. Flatten the masa into a large rectangle on the corn husk. Add about 2 large tablespoons full of filling down the middle of the masa rectangle in a strip. Roll the tamale up and repeat until all tamales are made. Steam the tamales in a steamer for about 1 1/2 hours.

Per tamale: 197 calories · 12 g fat · 2 g saturated fat · 52% calories from fat · 0 mg cholesterol · 7 g protein · 19 g carbohydrate · 2 g sugar · 3 g fiber · 700 mg sodium · 144 mg calcium · 3 mg iron · 6 mg vitamin C · 83 mcg beta-carotene · 2 mg vitamin E

VEGAN POLENTA WITH BALSAMIC GLAZED ONIONS

Muse, Corcoran Gallery of Art, Washington, District of Columbia

MAKES 6 SERVINGS

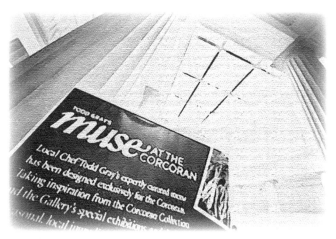

Since 1869 until it closed in October 2014, the Corcoran Gallery of Art, a block from the White House, has shown the best of American art. One hundred forty-three years later, it launched a new tradition, whipping up a vegan brunch in the middle of the ground-floor gallery. This popular dish will still color your day just right.

POLENTA

5 cups water	1 teaspoon salt
2 tablespoons extra-virgin olive oil	1 cup cornmeal

BALSAMIC GLAZED ONIONS

3 large purple onions	1/4 cup balsamic vinegar
1/4 cup extra-virgin olive oil	1 tablespoon maple syrup
1 teaspoon salt	6 fresh thyme sprigs, for garnish
1 tablespoon fresh thyme	

For polenta: In a medium stockpot, bring the water, olive oil, and salt to a rolling boil over high heat. Slowly whisk in the cornmeal so it does not form lumps. Reduce the heat to low and whisk the polenta often for 40 minutes or until it is tender and no longer grainy, taking care to scrape the bottom and sides of the pan while stirring.

For balsamic glazed onions: Preheat a cast iron pan over high heat until wisps of smoke rise from the surface.

Peel the onions, removing the root end and slicing the onions horizontally through the middle to form half-inch thick rings. Set aside 1 cup of sliced onions and chop those coarsely. Toss all onions in a large mixing bowl with the olive oil, salt, and thyme.

Place onions in pan and sear on high heat, stirring until a quarter of the onions form a browned skin. Turn heat to low and cook for 20 to 25 minutes, stirring every few minutes.

Meanwhile, whisk balsamic vinegar and maple syrup together. Pour over onions and cook over low heat, stirring constantly until a glaze forms on the onions, approximately 3 minutes.

Spread 2/3 cup of polenta on plate, swirling with the back of a spoon so that there's a slight well in the middle. Spoon 1/4 cup of onions into the middle of the polenta, then top with a generous spoonful of polenta. Garnish with a sprig of thyme.

Per serving (1/6 of recipe): 263 calories · 14 g fat · 2 g saturated fat · 47% calories from fat · 0 mg cholesterol · 3 g protein · 31 g carbohydrate · 7 g sugar · 2 g fiber · 801 mg sodium · 29 mg calcium · 2 mg iron · 4 mg vitamin C · 37 mcg beta-carotene · 2 mg vitamin E

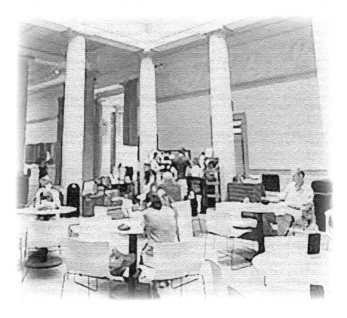

SPINACH TOFUCAKES

Mark's Kitchen, Takoma Park, Maryland

MAKES 4 SERVINGS

*I*n Takoma Park, Mark's Kitchen serves a loyal following who can't start their weekend without its healthy breakfast. The spinach tofucake is one of its signatures.

1 pound firm tofu
10 fresh spinach leaves, chopped
1 tablespoon breadcrumbs
1/4 red bell pepper, chopped
1/4 cup chopped green onion
1 teaspoon salt

1/2 teaspoon black pepper
1/4 cup sesame oil
1 teaspoon lemon juice (fresh is the best)
2 tablespoons soybean oil

OPTIONAL TOPPINGS

low-sodium soy sauce
chopped scallions

baby greens

Mix and crush the tofu and the spinach in a bowl. Add the bread crumbs, red bell pepper, green onion, salt, black pepper, sesame oil, and lemon juice. Form the mixture into 8 tofucakes, each approximately 1/2 inch thick and 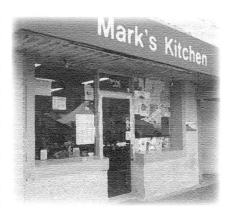 2 1/2 inches round. Pour a thin layer of soybean oil into a non-stick skillet and heat. Put the spinach tofucakes into the skillet in batches and fry from 3 to 4 minutes, until golden brown.

To serve, top with low-sodium soy sauce, chopped scallions, or baby greens, and serve over rice, if desired.

Per serving (1/4 of recipe): 304 calories · 27 g fat · 4 g saturated fat · 77% calories from fat · 0 mg cholesterol · 14 g protein · 6 g carbohydrate · 2 g sugar · 2 g fiber · 641 mg sodium · 338 mg calcium · 3 mg iron · 21 mg vitamin C · 1550 mcg beta-carotene · 1 mg vitamin E